Fourth Edition

Introduction to Audiology

A Review Manual

Frederick N. Martin
The University of Texas at Austin

Allyn and Bacon
Boston • London • Toronto • Sydney • Tokyo • Singapore

ISBN 0–205–19813–9

Printed in the United States of America

10   9   8   7   6   5   4   3   00   99   98

For Decibelle

Contents

DISORDERS DESCRIBED IN
CASE STUDIES

Acoustic Neuroma
Central Auditory Lesion
Collapsed Ear Canal
Congenital Hearing Loss
Méniére Disease
Noise-induced Hearing Loss
Otitis Media
Otosclerosis
Presbycusis
Pseudohypacusis-Bilateral
Pseudohypacusis-Unilateral
Serous Effusion

Preface

The purpose of this book is to help readers assess their knowledge of the basic concepts of audiology. Previous editions have been used by students in audiology classes, taking comprehensive examinations, or preparing for major tests such as the ASHA examination required of both audiologists and speech language-pathologists for the certificate of clinical competence.

Often students of audiology are not certain that they have learned the important materials from notes and textbooks. This book is designed to allow readers to test their knowledge by completing specific exercises based on facts and concepts that were learned from such sources as textbooks and lectures. There is evidence that learning and reinforcement of learning increase with writing, and so the user of this book is encouraged to fill in the appropriate spaces provided and then check the answers at the end of each unit or chapter. Wherever possible higher levels of learning are stressed, including application, synthesis, and generalization.

Part I contains twelve chapters whose contents parallel the Sixth Edition of *Introduction to Audiology*. Each chapter in this book, like its associated chapter in the text, deals with a specific area of audiology and attempts to utilize a variety of approaches to facilitate learning. In addition, twelve case studies are provided in Part II, each of which presents a patient's history and some audiometric data. On the basis of this information, the reader should be able to determine the type and degree of hearing loss, to discern the probable cause of the disorder, to explain why those conclusions were reached, and to make recommendations for proper case management.

Although this book is designed as a companion to *Introduction to Audiology*, its use is not necessarily tied to that book. Readers may use other primary sourcebooks or class notes to fill in any missing information. It is of the utmost importance for readers to diagnose their own knowledge deficiencies and correct them in the best and most expeditious way possible. The following pages will provide further direction on the best ways to use this book.

Frederick N. Martin

How to Use This Book

Part I—Review Chapters

This book is specifically designed *not* to provide new information or to teach new concepts but rather to assist readers in their efforts to monitor their own grasp of different aspects of audiology. When necessary, the reader should return to a textbook or lecture notes for needed information. Therefore, the study of each subject should be completed before a given chapter in this book is attempted. The purpose of this book is to augment, rather than substitute for, previous learning. The reader is expected to take the responsibility, with the aid of the workbook, for determining which areas require further review and study. If an incorrect answer remains misunderstood, the reader should return to a primary source for further explanation.

The table of contents lists the twelve chapters reviewed in this book and the twelve case studies. Some chapters contain more than one unit. Each unit should be approached in the same way, although the order in which the chapters are studied may be determined by the needs and wishes of the reader.

1. Read the paragraph providing the background material. It will be a very brief overview, and in some chapters, there will be more than one such paragraph, one for each unit. Each one covers a different aspect of the same subject. Certainly a single paragraph cannot provide all the information necessary to complete a review chapter or unit. Rather, it serves as an overview of a particular topic to reacquaint the reader with the subject at hand.
2. Read the stated objectives for each chapter or unit.
3. Complete the matching section to review the vocabulary of each subject.
4. Complete the outline for each chapter or unit. Write the letter that corresponds to a term from the right-hand column next to the appropriate number in the outline. The completed outline will provide a framework for review.
5. In those chapters with activities, write the answers directly in the book. This may entail additional matching, labeling, drawing graphs, or other activities.

6. Circle the correct answer to each multiple-choice question. Do not just assume that you will remember the correct answer.

When you have completed a chapter, check your answers against those at the end of each unit. If possible, do not peek at the answers until the entire chapter has been completed.

If you are uncertain of the definitions of some of the terms in the matching exercise, you should review a primary text. The Subject Index in *Introduction to Audiology* can be used to facilitate quick retrieval of the meanings of terms. The greater your working vocabulary, the better your chances for a successful understanding of audiology.

The purpose of the outline is to help you organize particular subjects. It is more than a mere matching exercise. You are forced to consider choices carefully because sometimes several items in the "Select from" column may be inserted into the outline in more than one place. Of course, if you wish to see the subject organization of a particular chapter without doing the outline, the answers may simply be copied from the back of the unit. The decision on whether to approach the outline with this strategy is left to the individual.

For many people, completing the chapters in this book is preparation for an examination. Once a chapter has been completed satisfactorily, or the reader recognizes weak points or corrects misconceptions, the sense of preparation can provide the sort of peace of mind that is always desirable before an examination. Those readers who do not do as well on a unit as they had hoped should be able to quickly identify areas of deficiency so that reviewing and learning the material can proceed logically.

Part II—Case Studies

Each theoretical case study is three pages long and represents a clinical diagnostic entity. Read the history statement on the first page. Then look at the audiogram, tympanogram, and other audiometric data on the second page. After you have reached your conclusions, fill in the appropriate spaces on the first page. Write down the probable etiology (cause) of each hearing disorder. Under "Case Management" write how you would handle the case, to whom a referral might be made, what might be said or written in a report, and so forth. Then write the reasons for your decisions. After this is done, check what you have written against the answers on the third page of the unit. If more information is required, read the appropriate chapter in *Introduction to Audiology* or another textbook. The conditions described in the case studies are listed in alphabetical order in the table of contents, but they are not referred to by page because it is your task to identify the particular disorder from the information provided. Listing the disorders by page numbers would reveal the correct diagnosis.

Part I

Review Chapters

C h a p t e r *1*

The Human Ear and Simple Tests of Hearing

UNIT A: THE FUNCTION OF THE EAR

Background

The ear is made up of three portions, the outer ear, the middle ear, and the inner ear. The outer ear is an acoustical chamber that picks up sounds from the environment and resonates at particular frequencies. At the end of the outer ear canal lies the eardrum membrane, which separates the outer ear from the middle ear. The middle ear, which continues the propagation of sound energy, functions in a primarily mechanical fashion, carrying vibrations to the inner ear. The inner ear is a hydromechanical system that transduces the energy it receives into electrical impulses; these impulses in turn transmit information about sound to the brain by way of the auditory nerve. The auditory system may be divided in a second, different way, one that separates the combined contributions of the outer and middle ears (called the *conductive* mechanism) from those of the inner ear and auditory nerve (the *sensorineural* mechanism). Damage to the conductive mechanism causes a conductive hearing loss, and damage to the sensorineural mechanism causes a sensorineural hearing loss.

Objectives

1. You should know and understand the terms in the matching exercise.
2. You should be able to fill in the outline, selecting items from the list provided.
3. You should be able to label the different parts of the auditory mechanism in Figure 1A-1.
4. You should be able to answer the multiple-choice questions on the function of the ear.
5. You should be able to complete the crossword puzzle.

Matching

Match the term from the column on the right with its definition.

Definition

1. ____ The sum of a combination of conductive and sensorineural hearing losses in the same ear

2. ____ Transmission of sound to the inner ear by vibration of the bones of the skull

3. ____ A tone presented to both ears simultaneously is perceived only in the ear in which it is louder

4. ____ Reduction in energy

5. ____ The course of sounds that are conducted to the inner ear by way of the outer and middle ear

6. ____ That portion of the hearing apparatus that converts mechanical energy to electrochemical energy

7. ____ The bony prominence behind the outer ear

8. ____ The most external portion of the hearing mechanism

9. ____ Loss of hearing because of damage to the inner ear or auditory nerve

10. ____ The sense that a sound is in the right or left ear

11. ____ The VIIIth cranial nerve connecting the inner ear with the brain

12. ____ The air-filled cavity behind the eardrum membrane that holds the three smallest bones of the body

13. ____ The loss of sound sensitivity because of damage to the outer or middle ear

14. ____ Reference to the sense of hearing

15. ____ The portion of the inner ear responsible for the hearing function

Term

a. Air conduction

b. Attenuation

c. Auditory

d. Auditory nerve

e. Bone conduction

f. Cochlea

g. Conductive hearing loss

h. Inner ear

i. Lateralization

j. Mastoid process

k. Middle ear

l. Mixed hearing loss

m. Outer ear

n. Sensorineural hearing loss

o. Stenger principle

Outline

The Human Ear

Outer Ear

1. _____

2. _____

3. _____

Middle Ear

4. _____

5. _____

6. _____

Inner Ear

7. _____

8. _____

Auditory Nerve

9. _____

Select From

A. Air-filled space with mucous membrane lining

B. Carries impulses to the brain

C. Eardrum membrane

D. External ear canal

E. Funnel-shaped structure

F. Open air-filled space

G. Snail-like structure

H. Tiniest bones in the body

I. Transducer

Activity

Label the items in Figure 1A-1. Select the terms from the list provided.

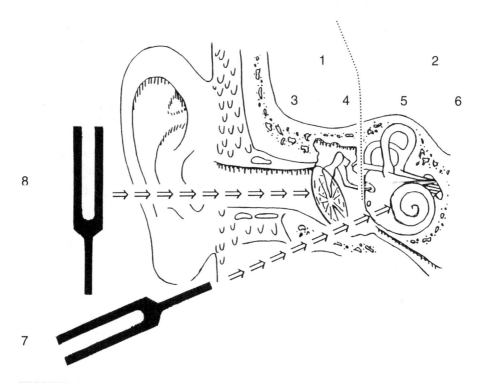

FIGURE 1A-1.   Coronal view of the ear.

Label	*Term*
1. _____	**A.** Air-conduction pathway
2. _____	**B.** Auditory nerve
3. _____	**C.** Bone-conduction pathway
4. _____	**D.** Conductive mechanism
5. _____	**E.** Inner ear
6. _____	**F.** Middle ear
7. _____	**G.** Outer ear
8. _____	**H.** Sensorineural mechanism

Multiple Choice

1. The air-conduction pathway is the
   a. outer ear, inner ear, auditory nerve, middle ear
   b. outer ear, middle ear
   c. outer ear, middle ear, inner ear, auditory nerve
   d. inner ear, auditory nerve

2. The bone-conduction pathway is the
   a. outer ear, inner ear, auditory nerve, middle ear
   b. outer ear, middle ear
   c. outer ear, middle ear, inner ear, auditory nerve
   d. inner ear, auditory nerve

3. When air conduction is impaired and bone conduction is normal, the interpretation is
   a. conductive hearing loss
   b. mixed hearing loss
   c. normal hearing
   d. sensorineural hearing loss

4. When air conduction is impaired and bone conduction is impaired to the same degree, the interpretation is
   a. conductive hearing loss
   b. mixed hearing loss
   c. normal hearing
   d. sensorineural hearing loss

5. When air conduction is normal and bone conduction is normal, the interpretation is
   a. conductive hearing loss
   b. mixed hearing loss
   c. normal hearing
   d. sensorineural hearing loss

6. When air conduction is impaired and bone conduction is impaired, but to a lesser degree, the interpretation is
   a. conductive hearing loss
   b. mixed hearing loss
   c. normal hearing
   d. sensorineural hearing loss

7. The conductive mechanism is comprised of
   a. outer ear and middle ear
   b. middle ear and inner ear
   c. inner ear and auditory nerve
   d. auditory nerve and outer ear

8. The sensorineural mechanism is comprised of
   a. outer ear and middle ear
   b. middle ear and inner ear
   c. inner ear and auditory nerve
   d. auditory nerve and outer ear

Crossword

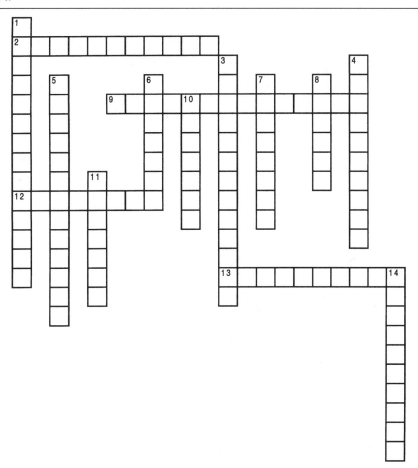

Across

2. Reduction of sound energy
9. The pathway of sound exclusive of the outer or middle ear (2 words)
12. Relating to the sense of hearing
13. The difference between the AC and BC thresholds (3 words)

Down

1. The impression that a sound is heard in the right or left ear
3. The type of hearing loss caused by damage to the inner ear or auditory nerve

4. The type of hearing loss caused by damage to the outer or middle ear
5. The pathway of sound including the entire hearing apparatus (2 words)
6. The way an organism is made
7. The most lateral, air-filled portion of the hearing mechanism (2 words)
8. The portion of the ear containing the three tiniest bones of the body
10. The transducer of the inner ear
11. The principle that states that a tone will be heard only in the ear in which it is louder
14. The way an organism functions

Answers—Unit A

Matching

1. l	**9.** n		
2. e	**10.** i		
3. o	**11.** d		
4. b	**12.** k		
5. a	**13.** g		
6. h	**14.** c		
7. j	**15.** f		
8. m			

Outline

1. D	**6.** H
2. E	**7.** G
3. F	**8.** I
4. A	**9.** B
5. C	

Activity

1. D	**5.** E
2. H	**6.** B
3. G	**7.** C
4. F	**8.** A

Multiple Choice

1. c	**5.** c
2. d	**6.** b
3. a	**7.** a
4. d	**8.** c

Crossword

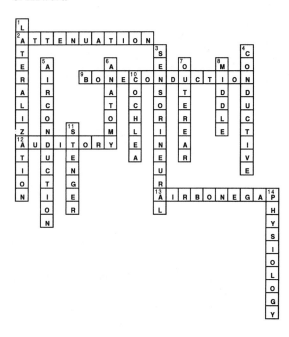

UNIT B: TUNING FORKS

Background

The tuning fork is a device borrowed from the profession of music by the medical profession. The tuning fork vibrates sinusoidally and comes closer to generating a pure tone than any other nonelectronic device. Most tuning-fork tests were developed by German otologists over a century ago and are still used by many practicing physicians. They have two primary values that justify their study: (1) They are of historical significance, and (2) they illustrate very well the relationships between air conduction (AC) and bone conduction (BC). The Rinne test compares a patient's hearing sensitivity by AC to BC; the Schwabach compares the patient's hearing by BC to normal (the examiner's) hearing; the Bing test checks for the occlusion effect, which should be absent in conductive hearing losses; the Weber test checks for lateralization in unilateral hearing losses. Tuning-fork tests are nonquantifiable, should be used to support audiometric data, and must be specified in terms of the frequency of the fork being used.

Objectives

1. You should know and understand the terms in the matching exercise.
2. You should be able to fill in the outline, selecting items from the list provided.
3. You should understand the four tuning-fork tests discussed in this unit in terms of performance and interpretation.
4. You should be able to answer the multiple-choice questions and understand the purpose and use of tuning forks.
5. You should be able to complete the crossword puzzle.

Matching

Match the term from the column on the right with its definition.

Definition

1. ___ The perception of increased loudness of a bone-conducted tone when the outer ear is occluded

2. ___ A tuning-fork test that compares the patient's hearing sensitivity by bone conduction with the examiner's

3. ___ Sounds that are conducted to the inner ear by vibration of the bones of the skull

4. ___ Attenuation of sounds as they pass through an abnormality of the outer ear or middle ear

5. ___ A metal instrument with a stem and two tines that is designed to vibrate at a single frequency

6. ___ A tone of only one frequency with no overtones

7. ___ A tuning-fork test that checks for the occlusion effect to determine the presence of conductive loss

8. ___ A tuning-fork test that compares hearing sensitivity presented by bone conduction to air conduction

9. ___ Conduction of sound to the inner ear by way of the outer and middle ear

10. ___ A tuning-fork test to determine whether a bone-conducted tone is heard in the right, left, or both ears

11. ___ Hearing loss produced by abnormality of the inner ear or auditory nerve

Term

a. Air conduction

b. Bing test

c. Bone conduction

d. Conductive hearing loss

e. Occlusion effect

f. Pure tone

g. Rinne test

h. Schwabach test

i. Sensorineural hearing loss

j. Tuning fork

k. Weber test

Outline

Tuning Fork Test

Rinne

1. _____

2. _____

3. _____

4. _____

5. _____

6. _____

Schwabach

7. _____

8. _____

9. _____

Bing

10. _____

11. _____

12. _____

14. _____

Weber

15. _____

16. _____

17. _____

18. _____

Select From

A. Absence of occlusion effect means conductive hearing loss

B. Compares AC sensitivity to BC

C. Compares patient's BC hearing to examiner's

D. Frequency must be specified

E. Heard in better ear in sensorineural hearing loss

F. Heard in poorer ear in conductive hearing loss

G. Louder by AC means normal or sensorineural loss

H. Louder by BC means conductive loss

I. Presence of OE means normal or sensorineural loss

J. Outer ear is occluded

K. Stem held against forehead

L. Stem held against mastoid

M. Tine held next to ear

Activity

Using Figure 1B-1, indicate the position in which a tuning fork should be held for each test.

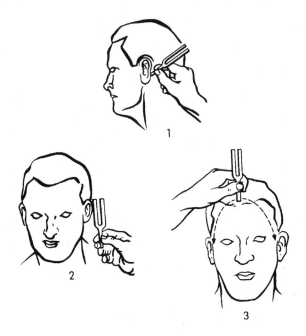

FIGURE 1B-l.   Tuning-fork positions for different tests.

Label

1. _____
2. _____
3. _____

Term

A. Bing test
B. Rinne test
C. Schwabach test
D. Weber test

Multiple Choice

1. One thing that should always be specified when reporting the results of tuning-fork tests is the
   a. frequency of the fork
   b. amplitude of the fork
   c. pressure of the fork against the head
   d. weight of the fork

2. A problem that tuning-fork tests have in common with any measurement made by bone conduction is that
   a. the nontest ear may hear the tone by bone conduction
   b. the patient may feel the vibrations
   c. pressure against the skull is a variable
   d. all of the above

3. In bilateral sensorineural hearing loss, the tuning-fork tests will theoretically show
   a. Bing negative: Rinne negative
   b. Bing positive: Rinne negative
   c. Bing negative: Rinne positive
   d. Bing positive: Rinne positive

4. A patient has a severe sensorineural hearing loss in the left ear and normal hearing in the right ear. Results on the Rinne test would be
   a. left positive: right positive
   b. left false negative: right positive
   c. left negative: right negative
   d. left false negative: right false positive

5. In unilateral conductive hearing loss, the Weber test will result in the sound being heard in the
   a. better ear
   b. both ears
   c. poorer ear
   d. neither ear

The next three questions are based on the proposition that your patient has a moderate conductive hearing loss in the left ear and a moderate sensorineural hearing loss in the right ear.

6. Results on the Rinne test should be
   a. positive right: positive left
   b. negative right: negative left
   c. positive right: negative left
   d. false negative right: negative left

7. If masking is used in the nontest ear, results on the Schwabach should be
   a. normal right: normal left
   b. diminished right: prolonged left
   c. prolonged right: diminished left
   d. normal right: diminished left

8. Results on the Bing test should be
   a. positive right: positive left
   b. negative right: negative left
   c. positive right: negative left
   d. negative right: positive left

9. A normal Schwabach can mean
   a. normal hearing or conductive hearing loss
   b. normal hearing or sensorineural hearing loss
   c. normal hearing or mixed hearing loss
   d. sensorineural hearing loss

Crossword

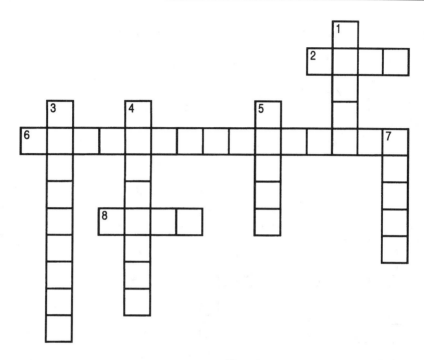

Across

2. A tuning-fork test utilizing the occlusion effect

6. The increased loudness of a bone-conducted tone when the opening to the ear is closed (2 words)

8. The portion of the tuning fork held by the examiner and pressed against the skull

Down

1. A tuning-fork test that compares the loudness of a tone by air conduction to bone conduction

3. A tuning-fork test that compares the examiner's hearing by bone conduction to the patient's

4. A signal of only one frequency (2 words)

5. A tuning-fork test involving lateralization

7. The portions of a tuning fork that vibrate actively

Answers—Unit B

Matching

1.	l	**7.**	b
2.	h	**8.**	g
3.	c	**9.**	a
4.	d	**10.**	k
5.	j	**11.**	i
6.	f		

Activity

1. A, B, C
2. B
3. D

Multiple Choice

1.	a	**6.**	d
2.	d	**7.**	b
3.	d	**8.**	c
4.	b	**9.**	a
5.	c		

Crossword

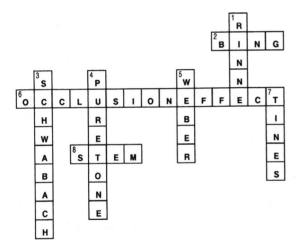

Chapter *2*

Sound and Its Measurement

Background

Sound is a wave disturbance that travels through any medium; humans are accustomed to hearing sound propagated through air. Three properties are necessary to produce sound waves: a force, a vibrating mass, and an elastic medium. Air molecules are the mass undergoing to-and-fro motion (vibration), and air itself has an elastic nature so that the molecules, in their vibratory motion, seem to be connected by "springs." Sound waves are produced by molecular vibration because of the pressure states that are created when molecules are packed closer together (compression states) or spread further apart (rarefaction states) than normal. As molecules undergo oscillation, successive compressions, followed by rarefactions, are passed along the line of particles at the speed of sound. Waves behaving with simple periodic oscillation are often called sine waves. These waves may be described in terms of how often they move from maximum rarefaction to maximum compression and then return to their point of origin: This is called the frequency of the wave. The intensity of a wave is the force that moves it to its maximum amplitude. The measurement unit for frequency is cycles per second (cps) or hertz (Hz). The measurement unit for intensity is the decibel (dB), a ratio between two sound pressures or two sound powers. Waves of different frequencies may combine to form interactions called complex waves. Frequency is interpreted psychologically as pitch, and intensity as loudness; different complex waveforms produce the quality or timbre of a sound.

Objectives

1. You should know and understand the terms in the matching exercise.
2. You should be able to fill in the outline, selecting items from the list provided.
3. You should be able to label the different parts of Figure 2-1 relating to sound waves.
4. You should be able to do the matching exercise on sound measurement units.
5. You should be able to answer the multiple-choice questions on the physics of sound.
6. You should be able to complete the crossword puzzle.

Matching 1

Match the term from the column on the right with its definition.

Definition

1. ___ The ability of a mass to return to its natural shape

2. ___ The exponent that tells the power to which a number is raised

3. ___ A unit of power

4. ___ A whole-number multiple of the fundamental of a complex wave

5. ___ The extent of the vibratory movement of a mass to the point furthest from its position of rest

6. ___ The portion of a sound wave where the molecules become less dense

7. ___ The amount of sound energy per unit of area

8. ___ The duration of one cycle of vibration

9. ___ A unit of expressing ratios in base 10 logarithms

10. ___ The waveform of a pure tone showing simple harmonic motion

11. ___ The difference between tones separated by a frequency ratio of 2:1

12. ___ The speed of a sound wave in a given direction

13. ___ A unit of pitch measurement

14. ___ The to-and-fro movements of a mass

15. ___ The distance between the same points on two successive cycles of a tone

16. ___ Reduction in amplitude to zero because of interaction of two tones 180 degrees out of phase

17. ___ The number of complete oscillations of a vibrating body per unit of time

Term

a. Amplitude

b. A periodic wave

c. Beats

d. Bel

e. Brownian motion

f. Cancellation

g. Component

h. Compression

i. Cosine wave

j. Damping

k. Difference tone

l. Dyne

m. Elasticity

n. Exponent

o. Force

p. Frequency

q. Fundamental frequency

r. Harmonic

s. Intensity

t. Logarithm

u. Mel

v. Microbar

w. Newton

x. Octave

y. Oscillation

z. Overtone

Definition

18. ____ A series of moving impulses set up by a vibration

19. ____ Progressive lessening in the amplitude of a vibrating body

20. ____ The impetus required to increase the velocity of a vibrating body

21. ____ Periodic variations of the amplitude of a tone caused by a second tone of slightly different frequency

22. ____ A unit of pressure equal to 1 Newton per meter square

23. ____ A logarithm

24. ____ A unit of force just sufficient to accelerate a mass of 1 gram at 1 cm per second squared

25. ____ A pressure equal to one-millionth of standard atmospheric pressure

26. ____ The lowest frequency of vibration in a complex wave

27. ____ The frequency of a tone produced by two tones of slightly different frequency

28. ____ A waveform that does not repeat itself over time

29. __ The relationship in time between two or more waves

30. ____ A force equal to 100,000 dynes

31. ____ The portion of a sound wave where molecules become more dense

32. ____ A pure tone constituent of a complex wave

33. ____ A unit of loudness measurement

34. ____ A waveform that repeats itself over time

35. ____ The constant colliding movement of molecules in a medium

36. ____ The unit of loudness level

(continued)

Term

aa. Pascal

ab. Period

ac. Periodic wave

ad. Phase

ae. Phon

af. Rarefaction

ag. Resonance

ah. Sinusoid

ai. Sone

aj. Velocity

ak. Watt

al. Wave

am. Wavelength

Definition

37. ___ The ability of a mass to vibrate at a particular frequency with minimum external force

38. ___ A sound wave representing simple harmonic motion that begins at 90 or 270 degrees

39. ___ Like a harmonic but numbered differently

Outline

Physics of Sound

Waves

1. _____

2. _____

3. _____

4. _____

Vibrations

5. _____

6. _____

Frequency

7. _____

8. _____

9. _____

10. _____

Intensity

11. _____

12. _____

13. _____

14. _____

Decibels

15. _____

16. _____

17. _____

Select From

A. Complex waves
B. Cycles per second
C. Decibel
D. Forced vibration
E. Fourier analysis
F. Free vibration
G. Hearing level
H. Hertz
I. Length effects
J. Longitudinal
K. Loudness
L. Mass effects
M. Pitch
N. Power
O. Pressure
P. Quality
Q. Sensation level
R. Sine
S. Sound-pressure level
T. Transverse
U. Work

Spectrum

18. _____

Psychological Acoustics

19. _____

20. _____

21. _____

Activity

In Figure 2-1 five parts of the sine wave are labeled. Each part may be referred to in two ways. Label each part appropriately.

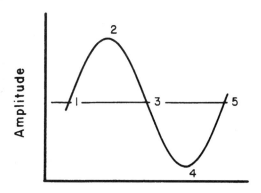

FIGURE 2-1.   Sine wave.

Label	*Term*
1. _____	**A.** Maximum amplitude
_____	**B.** 90°
2. _____	**C.** 180°
_____	**D.** 360°
3. _____	**E.** 270°
_____	**F.** Zero amplitude
4. _____	**G.** 0°
_____	
5. _____	

Matching 2

Match the measurement unit to each measurement below.

Measurement	**Unit**

Acceleration

1. _____

2. _____

Area

3. _____

4. _____

Force

5. _____

6. _____

Intensity

7. _____

8. _____

Length

9. _____

10. _____

Mass

11. _____

12. _____

Power

13. _____

14. _____

15. _____

Pressure

16. _____

17. _____

18. _____

Unit

A. Centimeter (cm)
B. Centimeter per second (cm/s)
C. Centimeter per second squared (cm/s^2)
D. Centimeter squared (cm^2)
E. Dyne (dyn)
F. Dyne per centimeter squared (dyn/cm^2)
G. Erg (e)
H. Ergs per second (e/s)
I. Gram (g)
J. Joule (J)
K. Joules per second (J/s)
L. Kilogram (kg)
M. Meter (m)
N. Meters per second (m/s)
O. Meters per second squared (m/s^2)
P. Meter squared (m^2)
Q. Newton (N)
R. Newton per meter squared (N/m^2)
S. Pascal (Pa)
T. Watt (w)
U. Watt per centimeter squared (w/cm^2)
V. Watt per meter squared (w/m^2)

Velocity

19. _____

20. _____

Work

21. _____

22. _____

Multiple Choice

1. Sound intensity
   a. decreases linearly as a function of distance from the source
   b. decreases inversely as a function of the square of the distance from the source
   c. is unaffected by the distance from the source
   d. is the same in fluid as in gas

2. Wavelength is
   a. sound velocity divided by frequency
   b. sound frequency divided by velocity
   c. frequency divided by a constant
   d. determined by intensity

3. If the fifth harmonic of a sound is 500 Hz, the fundamental frequency is
   a. indeterminable from the above information
   b. determined by wavelength
   c. 250 Hz
   d. 100 Hz

4. The period of a 100-Hz tone is
   a. 1/1000 sec
   b. 1/100 sec
   c. 1/10 sec
   d. 1 sec

5. Acceleration is
   a. the same as velocity
   b. the same as speed
   c. velocity divided by time
   d. 0 to 60 mph in 9 sec

6. When the expression *sound-pressure level* is used, this means that the reference is
   a. 10^{-16} watt/cm^2
   b. 0.002 dyn/cm^2
   c. 20 Pascals
   d. 20 micropascals

7. When the expression *intensity level* (IL) is used, this means that the reference is not
   a. 10^{-16} watt/cm^2
   b. 10^{-12} watt/m^2
   c. in decibels
   d. 0.0002 dyn/cm^2

8. The unit of measurement for pitch is the
   a. sone
   b. phon
   c. hertz
   d. mel

9. The SPL of a sound with a pressure output of 200 micropascals is
   a. 10 dB
   b. 20 dB
   c. 30 dB
   d. 40 dB

10. The IL of a sound is 50 dB. Its intensity output is
    a. 10^{-7} watt/m^2
    b. 100 dB
    c. 20 micropascals
    d. 0.0002 dyn/cm^2

11. The velocity of sound in air is said to be
    a. 20 mph
    b. 1,130 ft/sec
    c. 5,286 ft/sec
    d. faster than a speeding bullet

12. Masking may take place when
    a. the masker precedes the maskee
    b. the maskee precedes the masker
    c. the masker and maskee coexist in time
    d. all of the above

13. At its resonant frequency, a mass vibrates
    a. with the least amount of applied energy
    b. with the greatest amount of applied energy
    c. at its least possible amplitude
    d. as a free vibration

14. The condition in which air molecules are packed most tightly together is called the
    a. resonant frequency
    b. rarefaction
    c. sine wave
    d. compression

15. The quality of a sound is also called its
    a. phase
    b. pure tone
    c. timbre
    d. resonance

16. In the propagation of sound, as air molecules are moved further from each other they are said to be
    a. condensed
    b. compressed
    c. inert
    d. rarefied

17. The log of 1 is
    a. 0
    b. 1
    c. 2
    d. 3

18. Sounds we hear may be the result of
    a. incident waves
    b. reflected waves
    c. composite waves
    d. all of the above

19. The velocity of sound is
    a. unaffected by the medium
    b. greater in denser media
    c. greater in less dense media
    d. none of the above

20. The joule is a unit of
   a. work
   b. power
   c. intensity
   d. frequency

21. The unit of measurement in equal loudness contours is
   a. mel
   b. sone
   c. decibel
   d. phon

Crossword

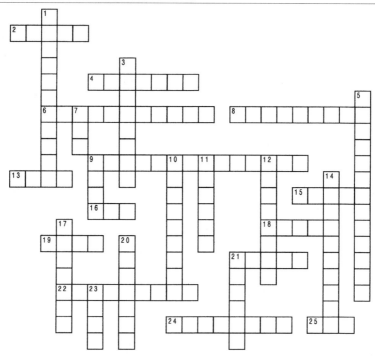

Across

2. Periodic variations in the amplitudes of two tones that are close in frequency
4. Analysis that breaks a complex wave into its components
6. Portion of a sound wave where molecules are condensed
8. Ability of a mass to vibrate at a frequency requiring the least external force
9. Number of decibels above the threshold of an individual (2 words)
13. Unit of force
15. Relationship in time between two or more waves
16. A unit of work
18. Complete sequence of events of a sine wave
19. Unit of loudness measurement
21. Subjective impression of the highness or lowness of a sound
22. Maximum extent of vibratory movement
24. A whole-number multiple of the fundamental frequency of a complex wave
25. Unit of impedance

Down

1. Portion of a sound wave where molecules are less densely packed
3. A tone containing no harmonics (2 words)
5. A short-term echo
7. Unit of pitch measurement
9. Kind of wave showing simple harmonic motion
10. Lowest intensity at which a sound can be heard
11. Difference between tones separated by a frequency ratio 2:1
12. The speed of sound
14. Distance between identical points on two successive waves
17. Concentration of energy in the spectrum of a vowel
20. Ratio between two sound pressures or two sound powers
21. Duration of one cycle of vibration
23. Unit of loudness level

Answers

Matching 1

1. m	**12.** aj	**23.** n	**34.** ac
2. t	**13.** u	**24.** l	**35.** e
3. ak	**14.** y	**25.** v	**36.** ae
4. r	**15.** am	**26.** q	**37.** ag
5. a	**16.** f	**27.** k	**38.** i
6. af	**17.** p	**28.** b	**39.** z
7. s	**18.** al	**29.** ad	
8. ab	**19.** j	**30.** w	
9. d	**20.** o	**31.** h	
10. ah	**21.** c	**32.** g	
11. x	**22.** aa	**33.** ai	

Outline

1. A	**12.** N
2. J	**13.** 0
3. R	**14.** U
4. T	**15.** G
5. D	**16.** Q
6. F	**17.** S
7. B	**18.** E
8. H	**19.** K
9. I	**20.** M
10. L	**21.** P
11. C	

Activity

1. F
G
2. A
B
3. C
F
4. A
E
5. D
F

Matching 2

1. C	**12.** L
2. O	**13.** H
3. D	**14.** K
4. P	**15.** T
5. E	**16.** F
6. Q	**17.** R
7. U	**18.** S
8. V	**19.** B
9. A	**20.** N
10. M	**21.** G
11. I	**22.** J

Crossword

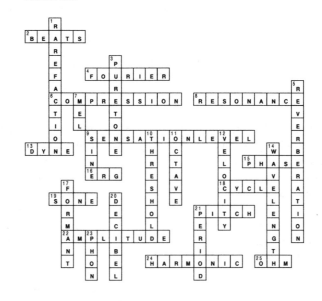

Multiple Choice

1. b	**12.** d
2. a	**13.** a
3. d	**14.** d
4. b	**15.** c
5. c	**16.** d
6. d	**17.** a
7. d	**18.** d
8. d	**19.** b
9. b	**20.** a
10. a	**21.** d
11. b	

Chapter 3

Pure-Tone Audiometry

UNIT A: TESTS WITH PURE TONES

Background

The pure-tone audiogram is a graph that depicts a patient's thresholds of audibility for a series of pure tones. The graph is arranged so that intensity (in dB HL) is shown on the ordinate: The lower on the graph, the greater the intensity—with 0-dB HL near the top and 110-dB HL near the bottom. Frequency is shown on the abscissa: The further to the right, the higher the frequency—with 125 Hz near the left and 8000 Hz near the right. A patient's threshold is measured for each ear by air conduction (AC) with the use of earphones. Threshold is also measured by bone conduction (BC), using a special oscillator. As each threshold is measured, the appropriate symbol is placed on the vertical line indicating the frequency tested where it intersects the horizontal line showing the intensity required to reach threshold. A red O is used for the right ear and a blue X for the left ear. The AC threshold for each frequency reveals the total amount of hearing loss; the BC threshold reveals the amount of hearing loss (if any) that is sensorineural; the amount by which hearing by AC is poorer than hearing by BC reveals any conductive component, or air-bone gap (ABG), of the hearing loss. AC symbols should be connected with a solid line, and BC symbols should either not be connected or be connected with a dashed line. Audiograms may show normal hearing, conductive hearing loss, sensorineural hearing loss, or mixed hearing loss.

Objectives

1. You should know and understand the terms in the matching exercise.
2. You should be able to fill in the outline, selecting items from the list provided.
3. You should memorize the symbols used in plotting an audiogram, including those for right and left ear air conduction and bone conduction. You should also know the symbols to use when masking is used in the opposite ear.
4. You should be able to draw an audiogram based on a patient's thresholds for air conduction and bone conduction.
5. You should be able to interpret audiograms in terms of the type and degree of hearing loss.
6. You should be able to answer the multiple-choice questions and understand the purpose and use of the audiogram.
7. You should be able to complete the crossword puzzle.

Matching

Match the term from the column on the right with its definition.

Definition

1. ____ The horizontal line on an audiogram or other graph

2. ____ A device for determining the thresholds of hearing

3. ____ The testing of hearing by specially programmed computer-driven audiometers

4. ____ Measurement made of hearing sensitivity by using earphones

5. ____ Failure of a patient to respond to a stimulus that has been heard

6. ____ The average of a patient's thresholds obtained at 500, 1000, and 2000 Hz in each ear audiometry

7. ____ The level at which a stimulus is barely perceptible 50 percent of the time

8. ____ Measurement made that tests hearing sensitivity exclusive of the outer and middle ears

Term

a. Abscissa

b. Air-bone gap

c. Air conduction

d. Audiogram

e. Audiometer

f. Békésy audiometry

g. Bone conduction

h. Computerized audiometry

i. Ordinate

j. False negative

k. False positive

l. Pure-tone average

m. Threshold

Definition

9. ____ The amount of sound energy (in decibels) by which the air-conduction threshold exceeds the bone-conduction threshold

10. ____ A graph representing hearing sensitivity (in decibels) as a function of frequency

11. ____ A response during testing when no stimulus has been presented or was presented below the hearing threshold of the subject

12. ____ Testing hearing by having subjects track their own thresholds

13. ____ The vertical line on an audiogram or other graph

Outline

Audiogram Interpretation

The Graph

Abscissa

1. _____

Ordinate

2. _____

3. _____

4. _____

Code Color

Right Ear

5. _____

Left Ear

6. _____

Audiogram Types

Normal Hearing

7. _____

(continued)

Select From

A. AC threshold

B. Blue

C. BC threshold

D. Equal amount of loss for AC and BC

E. 15 dB or less for AC and BC

F. Frequency

G. Greater hearing loss by AC than by BC

H. Hearing loss by AC, Normal hearing by BC

I. Intensity in dB HL

J. Red

K. O (red)

L. Δ (red)

M. < (red)

N. [(red)

O. X (blue)

P. □ (blue)

Q. > (blue)

R.] (blue)

Audiogram Interpretation

Conductive Hearing Loss

  8. _____

Sensorineural Hearing Loss

  9. _____

Mixed Hearing Loss

10. _____

Symbols

Right Ear AC

11. _____ (unmasked)

12. _____ (masked)

Right Ear BC

13. _____ (unmasked)

14. _____ (masked)

Left Ear AC

15. _____ (unmasked)

16. _____ (masked)

Left Ear BC

17. _____ (unmasked)

18. _____ (masked)

Activity

Given the four sets of audiometric data below, draw the audiograms that follow (Figures 3A-1 to 3A-4), illustrating four basic conditions. Use the symbol indicating masking when an asterisk (*) is shown. Compare your graphs to the properly drawn audiograms (Figures 3A-5 to 3A-8) at the end of this unit.

TABLE 3A. Audiometric Data

	Right Ear						Left Ear					
	250	500	1000	2000	4000	8000	250	500	1000	2000	4000	8000
AC	40	40	35	40	45	40	35	45	40	40	50	45
BC	–5	0	5	10	0	—	0	0	5	5	0	—
AC	65	70	70	75	65	75	70	65	70	70	70	75
BC	25	30	35	40	50	—	25	30	40	50	55	—
AC	0	5	0	5	5	10	5	5	0	–5	0	5
BC	0	0	0	5	5	—	0	5	0	0	0	—
AC	25	30	35	45	50	60	30	40	45	50	60	55
BC	25	35	40	45	55	—	25	35	40	45	55	—

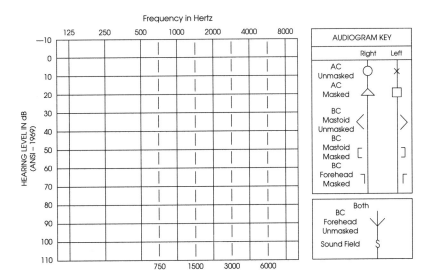

FIGURE 3A-1. Normal hearing.

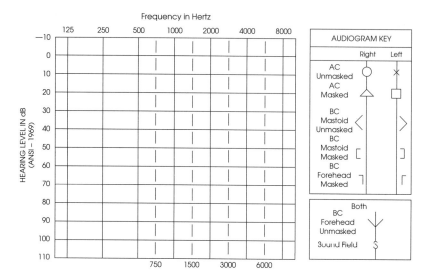

FIGURE 3A-2.   Conductive hearing loss.

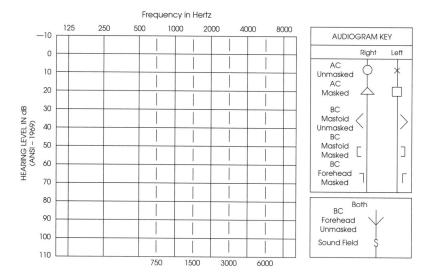

FIGURE 3A-3.   Sensorineural hearing loss.

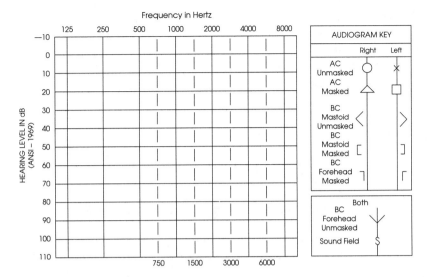

FIGURE 3A-4.   Mixed hearing loss.

Multiple Choice

1. The audiogram showing a conductive type of hearing loss will indicate
  a. impaired bone conduction, normal air conduction
  b. impaired air conduction, normal bone conduction
  c. impaired bone conduction, impaired air conduction
  d. normal bone conduction, normal air conduction

2. The audiogram showing a mixed type of hearing loss will indicate
  a. impaired bone conduction and an air-bone gap
  b. impaired air conduction and no air-bone gap
  c. impaired bone conduction and no air-bone gap
  d. normal bone conduction and an air-bone gap

3. The frequency range for bone conduction on most audiometers is
  a. 125–6000 Hz
  b. 250–8000 Hz
  c. 250–4000 Hz
  d. 125–8000 Hz

4. The maximum testable hearing level for bone conduction on an audiometer is usually
  a. the same as for air conduction
  b. greater than for air conduction
  c. less than for air conduction
  d. both a and c

5. The audiogram showing a sensorineural hearing loss will indicate
   a. impaired bone conduction and an air-bone gap
   b. impaired air conduction and no air-bone gap
   c. impaired bone conduction and normal air conduction
   d. normal bone conduction and an air-bone gap

6. The frequency range for air conduction on most audiometers is
   a. 125–6000 Hz
   b. 250–8000 Hz
   c. 250–4000 Hz
   d. 125–8000 Hz

7. For Figure 3A-4 at 500 Hz, the conductive portion of the hearing loss in the right ear is ___ dB
   a. 70
   b. 30
   c. 40
   d. 35

8. For Figure 3A-3 at 2000 Hz, the conductive portion of the hearing loss in the right ear is ___ dB
   a. 45
   b. 0
   c. –5
   d. 5

9. For Figure 3A-1 at 2000 Hz in the left ear, BC is 5 dB poorer than AC. This suggests
   a. normal variability and may be ignored
   b. a slight conductive hearing loss
   c. a slight sensorineural hearing loss
   d. a slight mixed hearing loss

10. For Figure 3A-2 at 4000 HZ in the left ear, the loss is
    a. completely conductive
    b. completely sensorineural
    c. partially mixed
    d. indeterminable

11. In determining the pure-tone average, the audiometric frequencies used are
    a. 250, 500, 1000 Hz
    b. 1000, 2000, 3000 Hz
    c. 500, 1000, 2000 Hz
    d. 250, 1000, 4000 Hz

12. An apparent sensorineural hearing loss with an air-bone gap only at 3000 and 4000 Hz is probably due to
    a. the occlusion effect
    b. cross-hearing by air conduction
    c. acoustic radiations from the bone-conduction vibrator
    d. acoustic radiations from the air-conduction receiver

13. If an audiogram is properly constructed, the distance across of one octave should be the same as the distance down of
    a. 5 dB
    b. 10 dB
    c. 15 dB
    d. 20 dB

14. Tactile responses to pure tones may be seen when stimuli are
    a. bone conduction only
    b. air conduction only
    c. bone conduction and air conduction
    d. sound field

Crossword

Across

3. Color used for plotting responses from the left ear
4. A means of expressing the energy of sound
6. Symbol used for plotting right-ear air-conduction thresholds
8. The 0-db reference found on an audiometer (2 words)
10. The vertical line of a graph
12. The number of complete vibrations of a body in a specified time

Down

1. The horizontal line of a graph
2. A combination of a conductive and sensorineural hearing loss
5. In audiology the least audible sound
7. Auditory signal of only one frequency (2 words)
8. Unit for measurement of frequency (abbr.)
9. Color used for plotting responses from the right ear
11. A graph representing hearing sensitivity as a function of frequency

Crossword

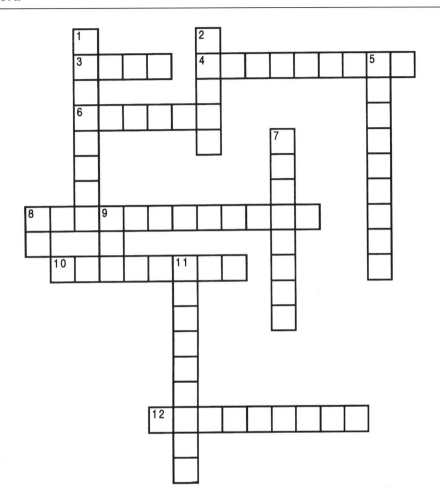

Answers—Unit A

Matching

1.	a	**8.**	g
2.	e	**9.**	b
3.	h	**10.**	d
4.	c	**11.**	k
5.	j	**12.**	f
6.	l	**13.**	i
7.	m		

Outline

1.	F	**10.**	G
2.	A	**11.**	K
3.	C	**12.**	L
4.	I	**13.**	M
5.	J	**14.**	N
6.	B	**15.**	O
7.	E	**16.**	P
8.	H	**17.**	Q
9.	D	**18.**	R

Multiple Choice

1.	b	**8.**	b
2.	a	**9.**	a
3.	c	**10.**	a
4.	c	**11.**	c
5.	b	**12.**	c
6.	d	**13.**	d
7.	c	**14.**	c

Crossword

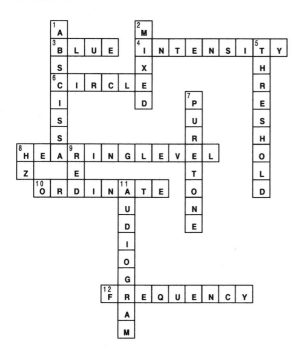

Activity

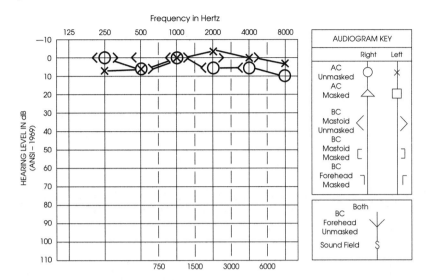

FIGURE 3A-5 Normal hearing.

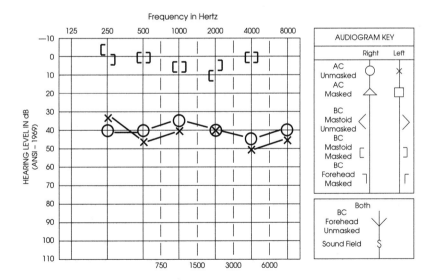

FIGURE 3A-6 Conductive hearing loss.

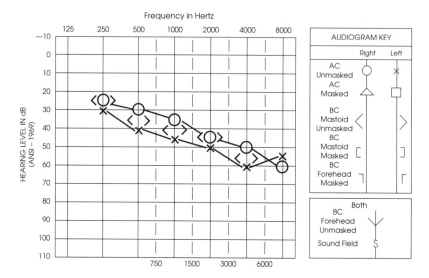

FIGURE 3A-7   Sensorineural hearing loss.

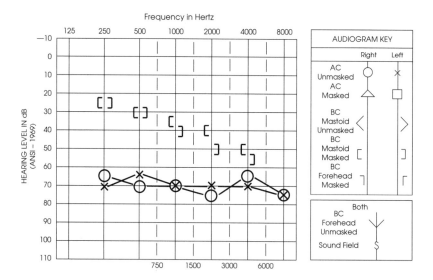

FIGURE 3A-8   Mixed hearing loss.

UNIT B: BONE CONDUCTION

Background

Bone-conduction tests may be performed with an oscillator from a pure-tone audiometer or the stem of a tuning fork pressed tightly against the skull. Pure-tone bone-conduction audiometry is performed to determine the sensorineural sensitivity of human hearing. Its purpose is to bypass the conductive mechanisms of the outer ear and middle ear and, by oscillating the skull, set the structures of the inner ear into vibration, resulting in neural transmission to the brain. The traveling wave set up in the inner ear by bone conduction is intended to stimulate the end organ of hearing. Therefore, whereas air-conduction tests measure the intensity of a signal required to reach a patient's threshold of audibility, including the entire auditory system, bone-conduction tests involve only the sensorineural structures of the inner ear and the pathways beyond. These principles are often violated by certain factors, and in many cases responses to bone conduction stimuli are modified by disorders of the outer ear and middle ear. Because both inner ears are embedded in the bones of the skull, it is virtually impossible to vibrate one without vibrating the other.

Objectives

1. You should know and understand the terms in the matching exercise.
2. You should be able to fill in the outline, selecting items from the list provided.
3. You should understand the principles of bone-conduction tests, why these tests are performed, and why they may not always achieve their objectives.
5. You should be able to answer the multiple-choice questions and grasp the fundamental concepts of bone conduction.
6. You should be able to complete the crossword puzzle.

Matching

Match the term from the column on the right with its definition.

Definition

1. ___ The mode of bone conduction involving the middle ear

2. ___ A test of lateralization performed by placing the bone-conduction vibrator on the forehead

3. ___ Introduction of noise into the nontest ear to eliminate cross-hearing

4. ___ The mode of bone conduction involving the outer ear

5. ___ The mode of bone conduction involving only the inner ear

6. ___ The increase in the loudness of bone-conducted tones that occurs when the ear is occluded

7. ___ A device used for calibrating the bone-conduction system of an audiometer

8. ___ Responses to bone-conducted stimuli that have been felt by the patient rather than heard

Term

a. Artificial mastoid

b. Audiometric Weber

c. Distortional

d. Inertial

e. Masking

f. Occlusion effect

g. Osseotympanic

h. Tactile

Outline

Bone Conduction

Outer-ear Effects

1. _____

2. _____

Middle-ear Effects

3. _____

4. _____

Select From

A. Affected by middle-ear conditions

B. Air pressure in middle ear

C. Distortion of temporal bone

D. Effects of covering the ear

E. Energy in outer ear canal

F. Poorer (higher) auditory threshold

G. Improved test reliability

H. Interaural attenuation

Inner-ear Effects

5. _____

6. _____

7. _____

8. _____

9. _____

Vibrator Placement

Mastoid Advantage

10. _____

Mastoid Disadvantages

11. _____

12. _____

13. _____

Forehead Advantages

14. _____

15. _____

Forehead Disadvantage

16. _____

Air-bone Relationships

17. _____

18. _____

Occlusion Effect

19. _____

Cross Hearing

20. _____

21. _____

Select From

I. Intertest variability

J. Less affected by vibrator pressure

K. Better (lower) auditory threshold

L. Masking

M. More affected by vibrator pressure

N. Ossicular chain impedance

O. Oval window release

P. Poor test reliability

Q. Round window release

R. Shearing of hair cells

S. Tactile response

T. Third window release

U. Tympanic membrane impedance

Multiple Choice

1. During bone-conduction testing, the low-frequency sounds appear louder when the ear is covered because of
   a. masking
   b. occlusion effect
   c. the Rinne effect
   d. cross-hearing

2. The mode of bone conduction affected by the outer ear is
   a. osseotympanic
   b. inertial
   c. distortional
   d. compressional

3. Interaural attenuation for bone conduction is generally considered to be ___ dB
   a. 0
   b. 25
   c. 50
   d. 75

4. Intertest variability may cause
   a. AC = BC
   b. AC > BC
   c. AC < BC
   d. all of the above

5. The occlusion effect is found at ___ Hz
   a. 250
   b. 250, 500
   c. 250, 500, 1000
   d. 250, 500, 1000, 2000

6. Testing bone conduction from the forehead requires ___ voltage to produce a response than testing from the mastoid
   a. more
   b. less
   c. the same

7. Forehead placement of the bone-conduction vibrator reduces the ___ mode of bone conduction
   a. inertial
   b. osseotympanic
   c. distortional
   d. compressional

8. The column of air in the external auditory meatus plays a large role in the ___ mode of bone conduction
   a. distortional
   b. osseotympanic
   c. inertial
   d. compressional

9. Advantages of testing bone conduction from the forehead over the mastoid include
   a. less effect of middle-ear disorders
   b. higher intensity required for threshold
   c. lower tactile thresholds
   d. greater interaural attenuation

10. To increase interaural attenuation when masking for bone conduction, one may use
    a. insert receivers
    b. standard receivers
    c. sound field
    d. a hearing aid

11. False air-bone gaps may not be produced by
    a. collapsing ear canals
    b. tactile bone-conduction responses
    c. contralateral bone-conduction responses
    d. distortional bone conduction

12. A profound bilateral sensorineural hearing loss might look like a mixed loss because
    a. cross-hearing has taken place
    b. bone-conduction responses were tactile
    c. ambient noise levels are too high
    d. improper masking was used

13. The mode of bone conduction affected by the inner ear is
    a. fractional
    b. unknown
    c. distortional
    d. osseotympanic

14. The impedance of the ossicular chain plays an important role in the ___ mode of bone conduction
    a. osseotympanic
    b. distortional
    c. inertial
    d. compressional

15. As frequency increases, the occlusion effect
   a. decreases
   b. increases
   c. remains unchanged
   d. decreases, then increases

16. In testing by bone conduction with the vibrator on the right mastoid process, the sound may be heard in
   a. the right ear
   b. the left ear
   c. both ears
   d. all of the above

Crossword

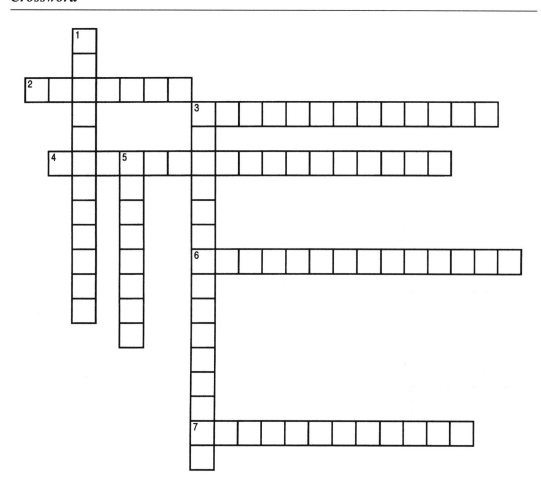

Across

2. The elevation of the threshold of sound caused by the introduction of a second sound

3. The mode of bone conduction associated with the outer ear

4. A device used for calibrating the bone-conduction system of any audiometer (2 words)

6. A device used during masking to increase interaural attenuation (2 words)

7. The nontest ear hearing a sound presented to the test ear (2 words)

Down

1. The mode of bone conduction associated with the inner ear

3. The increase in the loudness of a bone-conducted tone when the ear is occluded

5. The mode of bone conduction associated with the middle ear

Answers—Unit B

Matching

1.	d	**5.**	c
2.	b	**6.**	f
3.	e	**7.**	a
4.	g	**8.**	h

Outline

1.	E	**12.**	A
2.	U	**13.**	M
3.	N	**14.**	G
4.	B	**15.**	J
5.	C	**16.**	F
6.	R	**17.**	I
7.	O	**18.**	S
8.	Q	**19.**	D
9.	T	**20.**	H
10.	K	**21.**	L
11.	P		

Multiple Choice

1.	b	**9.**	a
2.	a	**10.**	a
3.	a	**11.**	d
4.	d	**12.**	b
5.	c	**13.**	c
6.	a	**14.**	c
7.	a	**15.**	a
8.	b	**16.**	d

Crossword

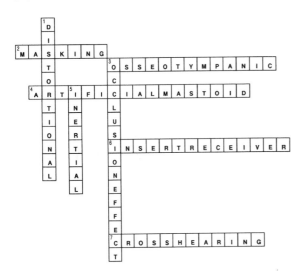

UNIT C: MASKING FOR PURE TONES

Background

Masking may be defined as the elevation of the threshold of a signal produced by a second signal concurrent with the first. The signal that is masked is called the maskee, and the signal that elevates the threshold is called the masker. In pure-tone audiometry the maskee is a pure tone and the masker is a noise. The noise should be specified in terms of its spectrum and its effectiveness in producing a threshold shift. Unless audiologists understand the effectiveness of the masking noise they use, they can do little more than work in the dark. Clinical masking must be applied whenever there is a danger that the threshold of the nontest ear may have been reached by cross-hearing. Cross-hearing for air conduction (AC) is generally considered to occur primarily by bone conduction (BC). The loss of intensity of a signal as it travels from the test ear earphone to the cochlea of the nontest ear is called interaural attenuation (IA). IA averages about 50–65 dB and varies with different people and with frequency. IA has never been reported to be less than 40 dB, which is a conservative figure to use when deciding on the need to mask. Since BC oscillations vibrate both cochleas with essentially equal force, the IA for BC is considered to be 0 dB. Masking for BC tests must, therefore, be carried out in every case or when masking might make a difference in diagnosis, that is, when there is an air-bone gap (ABG) in the test ear greater than 10 dB. If cross-hearing has taken place, the only way the threshold of the test ear can be determined is by the plateau method.

Objectives

1. You should know and understand the terms in the matching exercise.
2. You should be able to fill in the outline, selecting items from the list provided.
3. Based on the audiogram in Figure 3C-1, you should be able to determine the need to mask for each frequency for air conduction and bone conduction.
4. You should be able to determine the minimum amount of noise required to just mask out the nontest ear when necessary.
5. You should be able to label the parts of the masking plateau model in Figure 3C-2.
6. You should be able to answer the multiple-choice questions and grasp the fundamental concepts of masking.
7. You should be able to complete the crossword puzzle.

Matching

Match the term from the column on the right with its definition.

Definition

1. ___ A broad band noise containing approximately equal energy per cycle

2. ___ The level of noise that can be varied over a small range that does not alter the threshold of a sound presented to the opposite ear

3. ___ Introduction of noise into the nontest ear to eliminate cross-hearing

4. ___ The hearing of a sound in the ear opposite the one being tested

5. ___ The loss of energy of a sound as it travels from the test ear to the nontest ear

6. ___ A slight shift in threshold of a signal produced by a signal presented to the opposite ear that is not caused by peripheral (crossed) masking

7. ___ A band of frequencies surrounding a pure tone that is just wide enough to produce a threshold shift

8. ___ Masking of a stimulus produced by a noise in the nontest ear that crosses the skull and shifts the threshold of the test ear

9. ___ The lowest level of effective masking presented to the nontest ear during audiometry

10. ___ A broadband masking noise with energy concentrated in the low frequencies

11. ___ The minimum amount of noise required to mask out a signal in the same ear

12. ___ A restricted band of frequencies surrounding a particular frequency to be masked

13. ___ The highest level of noise that can be presented to one ear before it crosses the skull and masks the opposite ear

Term

a. Central masking

b. Complex noise

c. Critical band

d. Cross-hearing

e. Effective masking

f. Initial masking

g. Interaural attenuation

h. Masking

i. Maximum masking

j. Narrow-band noise

k. Overmasking

l. Plateau

m. Undermasking

n. White

Definition

14. ___ The result of insufficient noise presented to the nontest ear so that the threshold of the test ear cannot be determined

Outline

Masking for Pure Tones

The Need to Mask

For AC

   1. _____

For BC

   2. _____

   3. _____

Interaural Attenuation

For AC

   4. _____

For BC

   5. _____

The Plateau Components

   6. _____

   7. _____

   8. _____

   9. _____

  10. _____

Noise Types

  11. _____

  12. _____

  13. _____

  14. _____

  15. _____

Select From

A. ABG greater than 10 dB in test ear

B. $AC_{TE} - IA \geq BC_{NTE}$

C. Average 50 dB, Minimum 40 dB

D. Broadband

E. Complex

F. In all cases

G. Maximum masking

H. Minimum masking

I. Narrow-band

J. Overmasking

K. Pink

L. Plateau

M. Sawtooth

N. Undermasking

O. 0 dB

P. 250 Hz

Q. 500 Hz

R. 1000 Hz

Occlusion Effect—Frequencies

16. _____

17. _____

18. _____

Activity

In Table 3C indicate in the proper box whether masking is needed and the minimum amount of effective masking required to mask the nontest ear.

TABLE 3C   Masking for an Audiogram

| | Tone Right (Masking Left) | | | |
| | AC | | BC | |
Frequency	Masking needed?	Min em	Masking needed?	Min em
250				
500				
1000				
2000				
4000				

	Tone Left (Masking Right)			
250				
500				
1000				
2000				
4000				

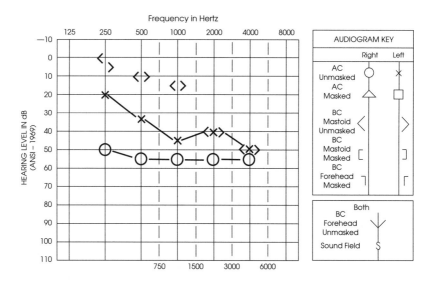

FIGURE 3C-1. An unmasked audiogram

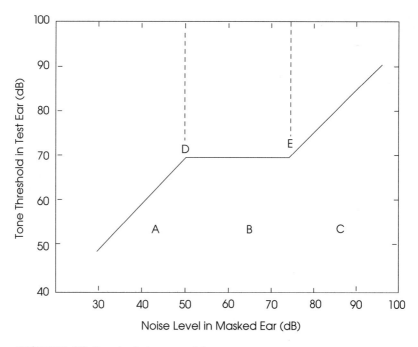

FIGURE 3C-2. A plateau model.

Label the five components of the plateau model.

A. _____   D. _____

B. _____   E. _____

C. _____

Multiple Choice

1. Cross-hearing is a possibility during pure-tone air conduction tests when
   a. $SRT_{TE} - 35$ dB $= BC_{NTE}$
   b. $ABG > 10$ dB
   c. $AC_{TE} - IA > BC_{NTE}$
   d. $AC_{TE} - BC_{NTE} = ABG$

2. The primary way by which cross-hearing for air conduction takes place is by
   a. skin conduction
   b. air conduction
   c. bone conduction
   d. cartilage conduction

3. The energy lost as sound travels from one ear to the other is called
   a. interaural attenuation
   b. cross-hearing
   c. contralateralization
   d. lateralization

4. The occlusion effect is tested during the ___ test.
   a. Bing
   b. Rinne
   c. Schwabach
   d. Weber

5. Minimum masking for bone conduction at 250 Hz is
   a. $EM = AC_{TE} + OE$
   b. $EM = AC_{NTE} + OE$
   c. $EM = AC_{TE} - IA$
   d. $EM = AC_{NTE} - IA$

6. Unmasked results on a patient with one normal ear and one ear with a total sensorineural loss show the poorer ear to have
   a. moderate conductive hearing loss
   b. moderate sensorineural hearing loss
   c. profound conductive hearing loss
   d. normal hearing

7. The audiometric Bing test determines the need for additional masking for
   a. bone conduction
   b. word recognition
   c. air conduction
   d. SRT

8. A predicted loss of sensitivity to an auditory stimulus in the presence of contralateral noise is called
   a. overmasking
   b. undermasking
   c. initial masking
   d. central masking

9. Masking is indicated for bone conduction when
   a. $ABG_{TE} > 10$ dB
   b. $ABG_{NTE} > 10$ dB
   c. $BC_{TE} - BC_{NTE} > 10$ dB
   d. $AC > 40$ dB

10. Overmasking is the greatest problem in
    a. bilateral conductive loss
    b. unilateral conductive loss
    c. bilateral sensorineural loss
    d. unilateral sensorineural loss

11. The most efficient kind of masking noise for pure-tone testing is
    a. narrow-band noise
    b. broadband noise
    c. high-pass filtered noise
    d. pink noise

12. The masking plateau becomes narrower as the
    a. bone-conduction threshold in the test ear gets lower (better)
    b. bone-conduction threshold in the test ear gets higher (poorer)
    c. interaural attenuation gets greater
    d. air-bone gap in the nontest ear gets larger

13. As the interaural attenuation increases, the masking plateau
    a. stays the same
    b. gets narrower
    c. gets wider
    d. changes in midfrequencies

14. Overmasking takes place for air conduction when
    a. $BC_{TE} + IA = EM$
    b. $BC_{TE} + IA - 10 dB = EM$
    c. $EM_{NTE} - ABG_{NTE} <$ True AC_{TE}
    d. $EM_{NTE} - ABG_{NTE} =$ True AC_{TE}

Crossword

Across

1. The signal used for masking
4. A practical calibration system for using masking noises (2 words)
6. A level that is unaffected by three consecutive increases of a masking noise
7. Excessive masking that produces a threshold shift in the test ear
8. The least amount of masking noise required to eliminate the nontest ear from test participation (2 words)

Down

1. The highest level of masking that can be used before overmasking takes place (2 words)
2. An insufficient amount of masking noise to allow determination of the threshold of a signal
3. The lowest practical noise level to use in beginning to mask (2 words)
5. The signal to be masked

Crossword

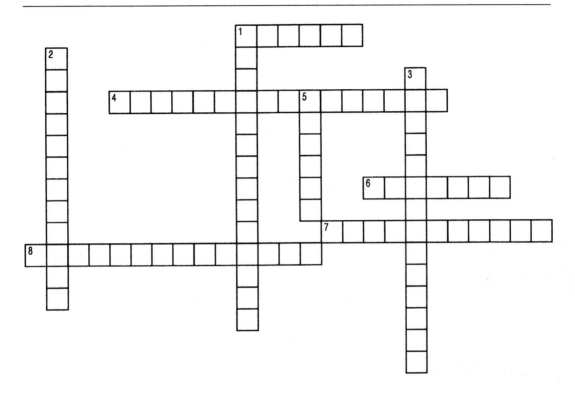

Answers—Unit C

Matching		*Outline*		*Activity*	*Multiple Choice*	

Matching

1. n   **8.** k
2. l   **9.** f
3. h   **10.** b
4. d   **11.** e
5. g   **12.** j
6. a   **13.** i
7. c   **14.** m

Outline

1. B   **10.** N
2. A   **11.** D
3. F   **12.** E
4. C   **13.** I
5. O   **14.** K
6. G   **15.** M
7. H   **16.** P
8. J   **17.** Q
9. L   **18.** R

Activity

Plateau

A. Undermasking
B. Plateau (range of EM in decibels)
C. Overmasking
D. Minimum masking
E. Maximum masking

Multiple Choice

1. c   **8.** d
2. c   **9.** a
3. a   **10.** a
4. a   **11.** a
5. b   **12.** a
6. a   **13.** c
7. a   **14.** a

Crossword

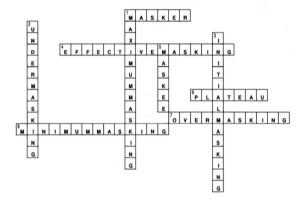

TABLE 3C   Audiogram with Masking

	Tone Right (Masking Left)			
	AC		BC	
Frequency	Masking needed?	Min em	Masking needed?	Min em
250	yes	20	yes	20 + OE
500	yes	35	yes	35 + OE
1000	yes	45	yes	45 + OE
2000	no	—	yes	40
4000	no	—	no	—

	Tone Left (Masking Right)			
250	no	—	yes	50 + OE
500	no	—	yes	55 +OE
1000	no	—	yes	55 + OE
2000	no	—	no	—
4000	no	—	no	—

Chapter 4

Speech Audiometry

UNIT A: SPEECH-HEARING TESTS

Background

Speech audiometry takes several forms and serves a number of useful purposes. Speech may be delivered by a monitored live voice or tape or disk recording through a speech audiometer to a patient by earphones or loudspeakers. Measurements can be made of a patient's threshold of audibility, word recognition, or most comfortable and uncomfortable listening levels. Speech audiometry is helpful in diagnosis of the type and degree of hearing impairment, in location of site of lesion, in rehabilitative measures such as selection of a hearing aid, and in determining the reliability of other tests such as the pure-tone audiogram.

Objectives

1. You should know and understand the terms in the matching exercise.
2. You should be able to fill in the outline, selecting items from the list provided.
3. You should be able to label the different parts of Figure 4A-1, showing the performance-intensity functions of speech stimuli.
4. You should be able to predict, within reason, speech test results from an audiogram.
5. You should be able to answer the multiple-choice questions and understand the uses and interpretations of speech audiometry.
6. You should be able to complete the crossword puzzle.

Matching

Match the term from the column on the right with its definition.

Definition

1. ___ The SPL at which speech becomes uncomfortably loud

2. ___ Introduction of speech through a microphone during speech audiometry

3. ___ A closed-message word-recognition test with emphasis on unvoiced consonants

4. ___ The highest word-recognition score obtainable from an individual regardless of sensation level

5. ___ The lowest level at which an individual can detect the presence of speech and recognize it as speech

6. ___ Monosyllabic words containing three phonemes each that are used in word-recognition tests

7. ___ A short phrase that precedes the stimulus word during speech audiometry

8. ___ A test that uses pictures to determine word recognition scores for children

9. ___ The difference (in decibels) between the threshold for speech and the level at which speech becomes uncomfortably loud

10. ___ Rapidly delivered, monotonous, and unemotional speech

11. ___ A device used for measurement of speech recognition thresholds and word-recognition scores

12. ___ A two-syllable word, used in speech audiometry, that has equal stress on both syllables

13. ___ A graph showing the percentage correct on word-recognition tests as a function of intensity

Term

a. California Consonant Test

b. Carrier phrase

c. Cold running speech

d. CNC words

e. Monitored live voice

f. Most comfortable loudness

g. PB Max

h. PI/PB function

i. PB word list

j. Range of comfortable loudness

k. Rhyme test

l. Rollover ratio

m. Speech audiometer

n. Speech-detection threshold

o. Speech-recognition threshold

p. Spondaic word

q. Uncomfortable loudness level

r. WIPI test

Definition

14. ___ A list of monosyllabic words used for determination of word-recognition scores

15. ___ PB Max – PB Min/PB Max

16. ___ The lowest intensity at which 50 percent of a list of spondees can be recognized

17. ___ The intensity (in dB HL) at which speech is judged to be most comfortably loud

18. ___ A closed-set word recognition test

Outline

Speech Audiometry

Speech-Detection Threshold

Purpose

1. _____

Material

2. _____

Speech-Recognition Threshold

Purposes

3. _____

4. _____

5. _____

6. _____

Materials

7. _____

8. _____

Word-Recognition Scores

Purposes

9. _____

10. _____

11. _____

Select From

A. CNC words
B. California Consonant Test
C. Cold running speech
D. Degree of hearing loss for speech
E. Detect presence of speech
F. Word recognition ability
G. 50 percent discrimination of speech
H. Selection of hearing aids
I. Intensity for greatest ease of listening
J. Intensity at which speech is just too loud
K. PB word lists
L. Reference level for WRS
M. Rhyme tests
N. Sentence tests
0. Site-of-lesion diagnosis
P. Spondaic words
Q. Synthetic sentence identification
R. Verify audiogram
S. WIPI test

Materials

12. _____

13. _____

14. _____

15. _____

16. _____

17. _____

18. _____

Most Comfortable Loudness

Purpose

19. _____

Material

20. _____

Uncomfortable Loudness

Purpose

21. _____

Material

22. _____

Activity

Label the four curves shown on the diagram that illustrate performance intensity functions. Select the terms from the list provided.

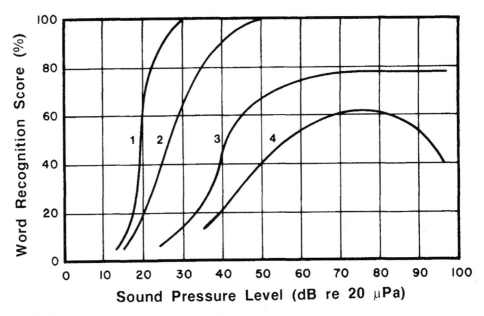

FIGURE 4A-l. Performance-intensity functions.

Label		*Term*
1. _____		**A.** Normal PB curve
2. _____		**B.** Normal spondee curve
3. _____		**C.** Rollover
4. _____		**D.** Word-recognition loss

Multiple Choice

Answer questions 1–7 based on the information contained in the audiogram in Figure 4A-2. If you are uncertain of the answer to question 1, check the answers at the end of this unit before proceeding with the questions.

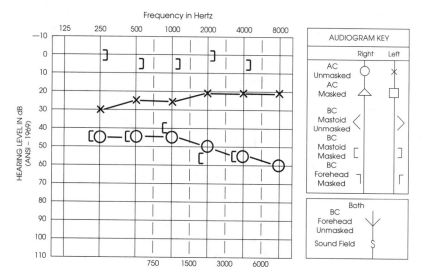

FIGURE 4A-2.   An audiogram.

1. The audiogram illustrates
   a. left mild conductive, right moderate conductive
   b. left mild sensorineural, right moderate sensorineural
   c. left mild conductive, right moderate sensorineural
   d. left moderate sensorineural, right mild conductive

2. A predicted SRT for the left ear is ___ dB HL
   a. 5
   b. 25
   c. 45
   d. 70

3. A predicted WRS for the left ear is ___ percent
   a. 6
   b. 40
   c. 80
   d. 100

4. A predicted MCL for the right ear is ___ dB HL
   a. 10
   b. 30
   c. 50
   d. 80

5. A predicted WRS for the right ear is ___ percent
   a. 2
   b. 30
   c. 78
   d. 100

6. A predicted UCL for the left ear is ___ dB HL
   a. 5
   b. 65
   c. 80
   d. 110

7. A predicted RCL (dynamic range) for the right ear is ___ dB
   a. 0
   b. 15
   c. 45
   d. 110

8. The relationship between SRT and SDT is usually
   a. SRT 10 dB lower (better) than SDT
   b. SRT 10 dB higher (poorer) than SDT
   c. SRT the same as SDT
   d. no relationship exists

9. Word-recognition scores are most commonly determined by using
   a. spondees
   b. PB word lists
   c. cold running speech
   d. WIPI

10. SRTs are usually measured with
   a. PB word lists
   b. spondaic words
   c. rhyming words
   d. nonsense words

11. The PI function for spondees is usually
   a. the same as for PBs
   b. more gradual than for PBs
   c. steeper than for PBs
   d. unreliable above 80 dB HL (hearing level)

12. The last word of the carrier phrase in word-recognition testing with PB word lists should
  a. strike zero on the volume units (VU) meter
  b. be equal in energy to the PB word
  c. be less intense than the PB word
  d. be more intense than the PB word

13. In audiograms showing sharply falling (in the higher frequencies) sensorineural hearing loss, the SRT is best predicted by the average of the thresholds at ___ Hz
  a. 500 and 1000
  b. 500, 1000, and 2000
  c. 500, 1000, 2000, and 3000
  d. 500, 1000, 2000, 3000, and 4000

14. The word-recognition score expected of a patient with a mild cochlear hearing loss is ___ percent
  a. 0
  b. 50
  c. 80
  d. 100

15. The word-recognition score expected of a patient with moderate conductive hearing loss is ___ percent
  a. 0
  b. 50
  c. 70
  d. 100

16. RCL(DR) is determined by the difference (in dB) between
  a. UCL and SRT
  b. UCL and MCL
  c. MCL and SRT
  d. UCL and PTA

17. The slope of the normal PI-PB function averages ___ percent per dB
  a. 2 1/2
  b. 5
  c. 10
  d. 12 1/2

18. PB MAX – PB MIN/PB MAX is the formula for
  a. percentage of hearing impairment
  b. rollover ratio
  c. word recognition score
  d. none of the above

Crossword

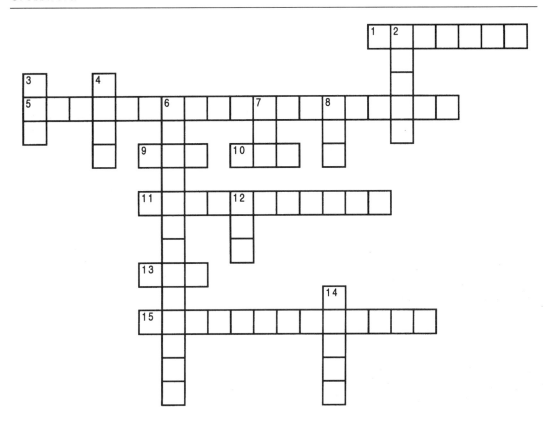

Across

1. A two-syllable word with equal stress on both syllables
5. A word-recognition test emphasizing high-frequency sounds (2 words)
9. Use of a microphone during speech audiometry (abbr.)
10. The tolerance limit for the intensity of speech (abbr.)
11. Speech that is rapid and unemotional (2 words)
13. the lowest intensity at which 50% of a list of words can be recognized (abbr.)
15. The words preceding the stimulus word during speech recognition testing (2 words)

Down

2. The highest word-recognition score obtainable regardless of intensity (2 words)
3. The intensity at which speech is found to be most desirable in terms of loudness (abbr.)
4. A closed-set word-recognition test for children (abbr.)
6. The relationship between PB Max and PB Min (2 words)
7. Stimuli used for word recognition that contain two consonants and a nucleus (abbr.)
8. The lowest level at which it is possible to be aware of speech (abbr.)
12. The difference (in dB) between the SRT and the UCL (abbr.)
14. A closed-set speech-recognition test in which the words differ by only one phoneme

Answers—Unit A

Matching		Outline		Activity	Multiple Choice	

Matching

1. q	**10.** c		
2. e	**11.** m		
3. a	**12.** p		
4. g	**13.** h		
5. n	**14.** i		
6. d	**15.** l		
7. b	**16.** o		
8. r	**17.** f		
9. j	**18.** k		

Outline

1. E	**12.** A
2. C	**13.** B
3. D	**14.** K
4. G	**15.** M
5. L	**16.** N
6. R	**17.** Q
7. C	**18.** S
8. P	**19.** I
9. F	**20.** C
10. H	**21.** J
11. O	**22.** C

Activity

1. B
2. A
3. D
4. C

Multiple Choice

1. c	**10.** b
2. b	**11.** c
3. d	**12.** a
4. d	**13.** a
5. c	**14.** c
6. c	**15.** d
7. c	**16.** a
8. b	**17.** a
9. b	**18.** b

Crossword

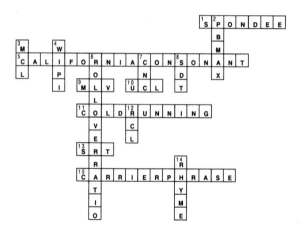

UNIT B: MASKING FOR SPEECH TESTS

Background

The possibility of cross-hearing during pure-tone tests is determined by comparing the air-conduction threshold of the test ear to the bone-conduction threshold of the nontest ear at the same frequency. This is done frequency by frequency. If the difference exceeds what may be the interaural attenuation for a given frequency, retesting must be done with masking in the nontest ear. The possibility of cross-hearing during speech audiometry is difficult to determine because the level of this complex broadband signal (speech) presented by air conduction to one ear must be compared to a pure-tone threshold obtained by bone conduction in the opposite ear. Since it cannot be known which of the frequencies in the nontest ear may contribute to cross-hearing of a speech signal, it is safest to compare to the lowest bone-conduction threshold at any frequency, although frequencies below 500 Hz probably contribute very little to the discrimination of speech. When the difference exceeds a conservative figure set for interaural attenuation (40 dB), masking should be applied to the nontest ear to render it temporarily incapable of responding. The use of effective masking (EM) appears to be the simplest way of approaching masking during speech recognition threshold and word-recognition testing. The problem of overmasking is greatest during word-recognition testing when there is a hearing loss in the masked ear (requiring a higher level of noise) and an air-bone gap in the test ear.

Objectives

1. You should know and understand the terms in the matching exercise.
2. You should be able to fill in the outline, selecting items from the list provided.
3. You should be able to determine the need to mask, based on an audiogram and unmasked speech thresholds for SRT and speech-recognition tests.
4. You should be able to determine the minimum amount of effective masking noise required to just mask out the nontest ear when necessary.
5. You should be able to determine when overmasking has taken place.
6. You should be able to answer the multiple-choice questions and grasp the fundamental concepts of masking for speech audiometry.
7. You should be able to complete the crossword puzzle.

Matching

Match the term from the column on the right with its definition.

Definition

1. ___ The ear opposite the one being tested

2. ___ The loss of energy of a (speech) sound as it travels from one ear to the other

3. ___ The lowest intensity at which approximately 50 percent of a group of spondees can be identified correctly

4. ___ The difference (in decibels) between the air-conduction and bone-conduction thresholds

5. ___ Insufficient noise to eliminate the nontest ear from participation in a speech test

6. ___ The greatest amount of noise that can be delivered to the nontest ear without overmasking

7. ___ The act of the nontest ear hearing a speech signal that is presented to the test ear

8. ___ A noise level high enough to lateralize from the nontest ear to the test ear and shift the threshold of the test ear

9. ___ The percentage of correctly identified items on a speech-recognition test

10. ___ The minimum amount of noise required to barely mask out a signal in the same ear

11. ___ The ear being examined on a hearing test

12. ___ The intensity at which a noise can be elevated three times without affecting the audibility of a speech signal in the test ear

13. ___ The least amount of masking noise required to eliminate the nontest ear from participation in a hearing test

14. ___ The elevation of the threshold of a signal produced by the introduction of a second signal

Term

a. Air-bone gap

b. Cross-hearing

c. Effective masking

d. Interaural attenuation

e. Masking

f. Maximum masking

g. Minimum masking

h. Nontest ear

i. Overmasking

j. PB hearing level

k. Plateau

l. Speech-recognition threshold

m. Word-recognition score

n. Test ear

o. Undermasking

Definition

15. ___ The hearing level at which an audiometer is set to carry out word-recognition testing with PB word lists

Outline

Masking for Speech Tests

The Need to Mask

For SRT

   1. _____

For WRS

   2. _____

Interaural Attenuation

   3. _____

   4. _____

Minimum EM for SRT

   5. _____

Minimum EM for WRS

   6. _____

Noise Type

   7. _____

Select From

A. Average 50 dB Minimum 40 dB

B. Broadband

C. Equal to SRT of NTE

D. $PBHL_{TE} - IA + ABG_{NTE}$

E. $PBHL_{TE} - IA \geq$ Lowest BC_{NTE}

F. $SRT_{TE} - IA \geq BC_{NTE}$

G. $SRT_{TE} -$ Lowest $BC_{NTE} \geq$ than 40 dB

Activity

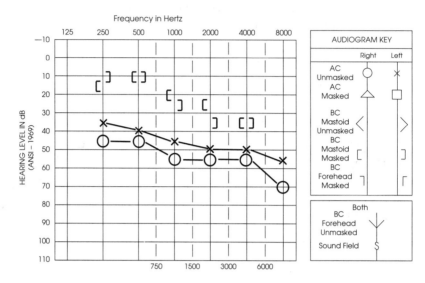

FIGURE 4B-l.   An audiogram.

In Table 4B, indicate in the proper box whether masking is needed for SRT and word recognition testing for each ear; also indicate the minimum amount of effective masking required to mask the nontest ear (if necessary). Assume that the word recognition test is done at 35 dB above the SRT.

TABLE 4B   Chart for masking.

	Speech Right (Masking Left)			Speech Left (Masking Right)	
Test	*Masking needed?*	*Min. EM*	*Test*	*Masking needed?*	*Min EM*
SRT-55 db			SRT-45 db		
SDS-?%			SDS-?%		

Multiple Choice

1. Of the following the most efficient masker to use during speech audiometry is
   a. narrowband noise
   b. broadband noise
   c. pure tone
   d. the identical signal presented to the test ear

2. It is always necessary to mask for word-recognition testing when
   a. there is an air-bone gap in the test ear greater than 25 dB
   b. the patient's interaural attenuation exceeds 50 dB
   c. the audiograms are asymmetrical
   d. masking was needed for SRT testing

3. The interaural attenuation for speech can be determined if
   a. there is an air-bone gap in the test ear
   b. the unmasked SRT is obtained by cross-hearing
   c. the test ear has a conductive hearing loss
   d. the test ear has a sensorineural hearing loss

4. For word-recognition tests, overmasking creates the greatest problem in
   a. bilateral mixed loss
   b. unilateral mixed loss
   c. bilateral sensorineural loss
   d. unilateral sensorineural loss

5. The need to mask during SRT testing is determined by comparing the
   a. SRT of the test ear to the pure-tone average of the nontest ear
   b. SRT of the test ear to the SRT of the nontest ear
   c. unmasked SRT to the opposite ear bone-conduction thresholds
   d. SRT of the test ear to the interaural attenuation

6. The need to mask during word-recognition testing is determined by comparing the
   a. hearing level of the test stimuli to the opposite ear bone-conduction thresholds
   b. SRT of the test ear to the interaural attenuation
   c. SRT of the test ear to the SRT of the nontest ear
   d. none of the above

7. Overmasking occurs during SRT testing when the
   a. test presentation level exceeds 95 dB
   b. interaural attenuation is greater than 60 dB
   c. test presentation level exceeds the SRT of the nontest ear
   d. effective masking level minus the patient's interaural attenuation equals or exceeds the bone-conduction thresholds of the test ear

8. Overmasking occurs during word-recognition testing when the
   a. test presentation level exceeds 95 dB
   b. interaural attenuation is greater than 60 dB
   c. test presentation level exceeds the SRT of the nontest ear
   d. effective masking level minus the patient's interaural attenuation meets or exceeds the bone-conduction thresholds of the test ear

9. The result of not masking during speech-recognition threshold testing may be that the
   a. SRT was obtained by bone conduction in the nontest ear
   b. SRT was obtained by air conduction in the nontest ear
   c. SRT was actually lower (better) than what was observed
   d. none of the above

10. The result of not masking during word-recognition testing may be that the
   a. word-recognition score is actually poorer than that which is observed
   b. nontest ear actually took the word-recognition test
   c. word-recognition test was actually taken by both ears
   d. all of the above

11. The result of overmasking during speech-recognition threshold testing may be that the
   a. SRT appears better than it truly is
   b. SRT appears worse than it truly is
   c. interaural attenuation is increased
   d. none of the above

12. The result of overmasking during word-recognition testing may be that the
   a. word-recognition score appears better than it truly is
   b. word-recognition score appears poorer than it truly is
   c. sensation level of the test is raised
   d. none of the above

13. When a patient's interaural attenuation is not known, it is safest to assume that it may be as little as
   a. 30 dB
   b. 40 dB
   c. 50 dB
   d. 60 dB

14. The air-bone gap of the masked ear must be added to minimum masking levels during speech-recognition testing because
   a. the conductive component of the loss attenuates the masking level
   b. the interaural attenuation is increased in conductive hearing losses
   c. masking is always needed when the test ear has a conductive hearing loss
   d. none of the above

15. Five decibels is often added to the usual sensation level for word recognition tests when masking is used to
    a. increase the interaural attenuation
    b. decrease the interaural attenuation
    c. account for cross-hearing
    d. offset central masking

16. If the interaural attenuation for speech can be determined to be greater than 40 dB, it is better to use the larger number to
    a. increase the likelihood of undermasking
    b. decrease the likelihood of undermasking
    c. decrease the likelihood of overmasking
    d. increase the likelihood of overmasking

17. Overmasking during SRT testing results in the
    a. threshold of the nontest ear getting higher (poorer)
    b. threshold of the nontest ear getting lower (better)
    c. threshold of the test ear getting higher (poorer)
    d. threshold of the test ear getting lower (better)

18. Overmasking during word recognition testing results in the word recognition score of the
    a. test ear getting higher
    b. test ear getting lower
    c. nontest ear getting higher
    d. nontest ear getting lower

19. One excellent means of minimizing the chances of undermasking or overmasking during speech audiometry is to
    a. test with insert receivers
    b. mask with insert receivers
    c. test and mask with insert receivers
    d. use standard earphones

Crossword

Across

2. The least amount of noise required to just mask out a speech signal (2 words)
5. The ear opposite the one being tested
7. Contralateralization (2 words)
8. The range between minimum and maximum masking
10. The highest level of masking permissible before overmasking takes place

Down

1. The difference between air- and bone-conducted thresholds (3 words)
3. A small threshold shift produced by masking that is not peripheral
4. The loss of energy of a sound as it travels from one ear to the other (abbr.)
6. The lowest amount of effective masking required to shift a threshold
9. Masking that is insufficient to eliminate the nontest ear

Crossword

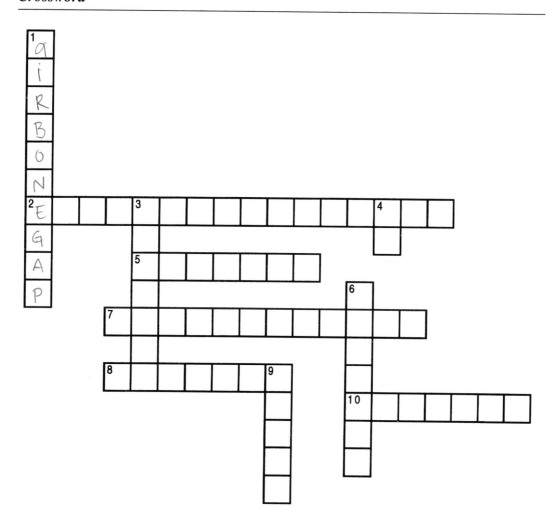

Down 1: A I R B O N E G A P

Across 2: E

Answers—Unit B

Matching

1.	h	**9.**	m
2.	d	**10.**	c
3.	l	**11.**	n
4.	a	**12.**	k
5.	o	**13.**	g
6.	f	**14.**	e
7.	b	**15.**	j
8.	i		

Outline

1.	F
2.	E
3.	A
4.	G
5.	C
6.	D
7.	B

Multiple Choice

1.	b	**11.**	b
2.	d	**12.**	b
3.	b	**13.**	b
4.	a	**14.**	a
5.	c	**15.**	d
6.	a	**16.**	c
7.	d	**17.**	c
8.	d	**18.**	b
9.	a	**19.**	c
10.	d		

Activity

TABLE 4B   Chart for masking.

	Speech Right (Masking Left)			Speech Left (Masking Right)	
Test	*Masking needed?*	*Min. EM*	*Test*	*Masking needed?*	*Min EM*
SRT-50 db	yes	45 db	SRT-45 db	no	—
WRS-Unknown	yes	75 db	WRS-Unknown	yes	70 db

Crossword

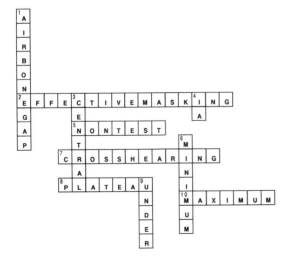

Chapter **5**

Auditory Tests for Site of Lesion

UNIT A: ACOUSTIC IMMITTANCE

Background

The word *immittance*, when applied to measurements at the tympanic membrane, is a combined form of the words *impedance* (the opposition to the flow of acoustic energy to the middle ear) and *admittance* (that acoustic energy passed by the tympanic membrane into the middle ear). It is a compromise in terminology. There is no disagreement, however, on the value that immittance has in the diagnosis of diseases in different parts of the auditory system. Three major tests can be carried out with modern electroacoustic immittance meters: (1) *static compliance*—a means of determining the degree of stiffness of the tympanic membrane and ossicular chain; (2) *tympanometry*—a measure of the compliance of the tympanic membrane with varying degrees of positive and negative pressure in the external auditory canal; (3) *the acoustic reflex threshold*—determination of the intensity of a sound required to contract the stapedius muscle when that sound is presented to the same ear as the probe, which senses tympanic membrane movement, or to the opposite ear. Immittance measures may indicate not only a middle-ear disorder but also its probable cause. Acoustic reflexes can help in determining the site of pathology in sensorineural losses, approximation of degree of hearing loss in noncooperative patients, facial nerve integrity, and more. No more valuable procedure has been added in recent years to the power of routine diagnostic audiology.

Objectives

1. You should know and understand the terms in the matching exercise.
2. You should be able to fill in the outline, selecting items from the list provided.
3. You should understand the implications of static immittance, including its possible weaknesses as a measurement of true tympanic membrane function.
4. You should be able to interpret the different types of tympanograms, know how they are obtained, and what they imply.
5. You should be able to sketch the different types of tympanograms.
6. You should know the implications of absent, elevated, and low sensation level acoustic reflex thresholds.
7. You should know some variations of the acoustic reflex test, including acoustic reflex decay, comparison of ipsilateral and contralateral acoustic reflex thresholds, and results of measurements made with different kinds of stimuli.
8. You should be able to answer the multiple-choice questions on acoustic immittance.
9. You should be able to complete the crossword puzzle.

Matching

Match the term from the column on the right with its definition.

Definition

1. ___ The lowest intensity at which a stimulus produces an acoustic reflex

2. _D_ The total contribution to impedance made by mass, stiffness, and frequency

3. _E_ The VIIth cranial nerve, which runs from the brain stem to the stapedial tendon

4. _K_ A small muscle whose insertion is in the neck of the stapes

5. _M_ Measurement of the pressure-compliance function of the eardrum membrane

6. _A_ Measurement of impedance or admittance of the eardrum membrane

7. ___ Contraction of the middle-ear muscles in response to sound

8. _B_ A graph representing the pressure-compliance function of the eardrum membrane

Term

a. Acoustic reflex

b. Acoustic reflex arc

c. ART

d. Compliance

e. Facial nerve

f. Immittance

g. Otoadmittance

h. Reactance

i. Reflex decay

j. Resistance

k. Stapedius

l. Tensor tympani

m. Tympanogram

n. Tympanometry

9. ___ A small muscle whose insertion is in the neck of the malleus

10. ___ The inverse of stiffness

11. ___ That portion of impedance that is independent of frequency

12. ___ The acceptance of acoustic energy from the eardrum membrane to the middle ear

13. ___ A decrease in the impedance of the eardrum membrane as a result of constant sound stimulation

14. ___ The ascending and descending pathways of the acoustic reflex

Outline

Acoustic Immittance

Equipment

1. _____

2. _____

3. _____

4. _____

5. _____

6. _____

7. _____

8. _____

9. _____

Static Compliance

10. _____

11. _____

12. _____

13. _____

Select From

A. Absent—conductive or severe sensorineural loss
B. Air pump
C. Balance meter
D. Compliance with TM loose
E. Compliance with TM tight
F. Contralateral earphone
G. Elevated—mild conductive loss
H. Low value—stiffness of TM and/or ossicular chain
I. Loudspeaker
J. Low SL—cochlear lesion
K. High value—interruption of ossicular chain
L. Manometer
M. Microphone
N. Oscillator
O. Potentiometer
P. Probe assembly
Q. Reflex decay—retrocochlear lesion

Acoustic Immittance

Tympanometry

14. _____

15. _____

16. _____

17. _____

18. _____

Acoustic Reflex Threshold

19. _____

20. _____

21. _____

22. _____

Select From

R. Type A—normal ME

S. Type B—fluid in ME

T. Type C—negative pressure in ME

U. Type A_S—stiffness of ossicular chain

V. Type A_D—very compliant TM

Activity

Sketch four different tympanograms on the following forms (Figures 5A-1 to 5A-4). Compare your graphs to the properly drawn tympanograms (Figures 5A-5 to 5A-8) at the end of this unit.

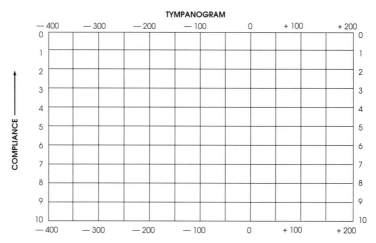

FIGURE 5A-l.   Type A.

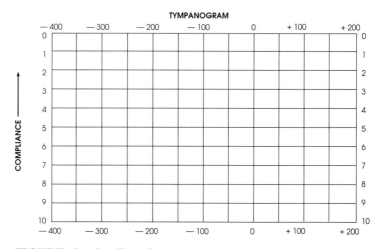

FIGURE 5A–2.   Type B.

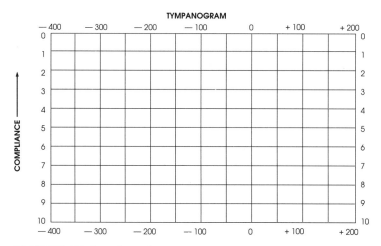

FIGURE 5A-3.   Type C.

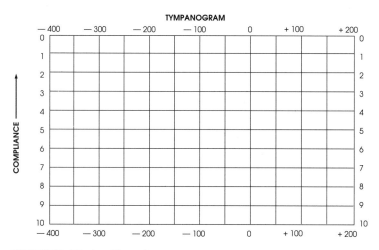

FIGURE 5A-4.   Type A$_S$.

Multiple Choice

1. Theoretically, a patient with otosclerosis should show
   a. normal tympanic membrane compliance
   b. higher than normal tympanic membrane compliance
   c. lower than normal tympanic membrane compliance
   d. fluctuating tympanic membrane compliance

2. Absence of an acoustic reflex is probable in
   a. conductive hearing loss
   b. profound sensorineural hearing loss
   c. facial nerve paralysis
   d. all of the above

3. A patient has a 40 dB hearing loss caused by otosclerosis in the left ear. Acoustic reflexes with contralateral stimulation would probably show
   a. absent right, absent left
   b. present right, present left
   c. present right, absent left
   d. absent right, present left

4. Type B tympanograms may be attributed to any of the following except
   a. otitis media
   b. impacted cerumen
   c. interrupted ossicular chain
   d. probe opening against canal wall

5. A retracted tympanic membrane should yield a tympanogram type
   a. A
   b. B
   c. C
   d. D

6. Of the following, the most likely tympanogram to occur in the presence of otosclerosis is
   a. A_S
   b. A_D
   c. B
   d. C

7. A measured increase in compliance of the tympanic membrane may result from
   a. interrupted ossicular chain
   b. middle-ear infection
   c. perforated tympanic membrane
   d. ceruminosis

8. An acoustic reflex at a sensation level below 55 dB suggests
   a. no pathology
   b. middle-ear pathology
   c. cochlear pathology
   d. auditory nerve pathology

9. The portion of the ear responsible for the stiffness component of impedance in the plane of the tympanic membrane is the
   a. tympanic membrane
   b. ossicular ligaments
   c. ossicular mass
   d. fluid load on the stapes

10. A tympanogram with no point of maximum compliance indicates the probable presence of
    a. Méniére disease
    b. otitis media
    c. broken incus
    d. otosclerosis

11. Theoretically an interrupted ossicular chain shows the tympanogram type
    a. A
    b. A_S
    c. A_D
    d. C

12. A tympanogram with maximum compliance at −200 daPa suggests
    a. normally aerated middle ear
    b. negative pressure in the middle ear
    c. positive pressure in the middle ear
    d. fluid in the middle ear

13. According to the impedance formula, early otosclerosis should result in an audiometric configuration that is
    a. basically flat
    b. worse in the high frequencies
    c. worse in the mid-frequencies
    d. worse in the low frequencies

14. A tympanogram with no point of maximum compliance could result from
    a. fluid in the middle ear
    b. negative pressure in the middle ear
    c. a normally aerated middle ear
    d. positive pressure in the middle ear

15. In the use of an immittance meter with probe in the right ear and the phone over the left ear, the contralateral acoustic reflex is designed to measure the
    a. Vth nerve left, reflex SL right
    b. recruitment right, decruitment left
    c. facial nerve left, reflex SL right
    d. facial nerve right, reflex SL left

16. Your patient has an intra-axial brain-stem lesion on the right side but normal hearing for pure tones in both ears. Acoustic reflex results should be as follows:
    a. Contralateral: present left, absent right
       Ipsilateral: present left, present right
    b. Contralateral: present right, present left
       Ipsilateral: absent right, present left
    c. Contralateral: absent right, absent left
       Ipsilateral: absent right, present left
    d. Contralateral: present right, present left
       Ipsilateral: absent right, absent left

17. Acoustic reflexes at 5-dB SL suggest
    a. retrocochlear lesion
    b. cochlear lesion
    c. conductive lesion
    d. pseudohypacusis

18. The tympanic membrane is maximally compliant when
    a. middle-ear pressure equals outer-ear pressure
    b. middle-ear pressure is less than outer-ear pressure
    c. middle-ear pressure is greater than outer-ear pressure
    d. all of the above

19. Reflex decay at 500, Hz to half amplitude within 10 seconds suggests
    a. pseudohypacusis
    b. conductive lesion
    c. cochlear lesion
    d. retrocochlear lesion

20. During measurements of static compliance, a patient's Cl reading is 5.0 cc. This suggests
    a. interrupted ossicular chain
    b. otosclerosis
    c. tympanic membrane perforation
    d. otitis media

21. The component of impedance unrelated to frequency is
   a. resistance
   b. mass
   c. stiffness
   d. pi

22. Present in the contralateral acoustic reflex pathway but absent in the ipsilateral acoustic reflex pathway are the
   a. cochlear nuclei
   b. decussations
   c. auditory nerves
   d. superior olivary complexes

Crossword

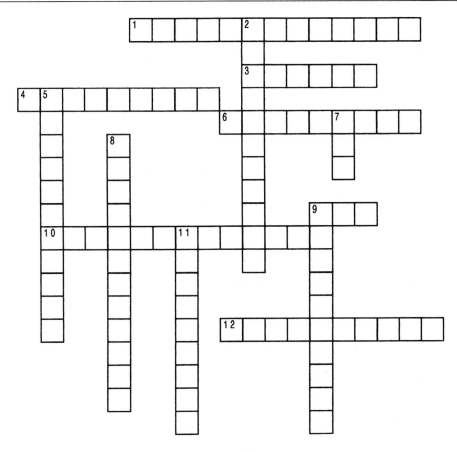

Across

1. A muscle that inserts into the neck of the malleus (2 words)
3. The VIIth cranial nerve that stimulates the stapedius muscle
4. The muscle that inserts into the neck of the stapes
6. That portion of impedance that relates both mass and stiffness to frequency
9. A signal that causes stapedial muscle contraction (abbr.)
10. Measurement of a sound that is admitted to the middle ear from the tympanic membrane
12. A term describing both impedance and admittance

Down

2. The rate at which the stapedium muscle relaxes after contracting in response to sound (2 words)
5. A graph that depicts tympanic membrane immitance as a function of air pressure
7. The lowest sound intensity that causes contraction of the middle-ear muscles (abbr.)
8. The compliance of the tympanic membrane as a function of air pressure against the TM
9. The portion of the impedance formula that is independent of frequency
11. The opposition to the flow of energy

Answers—Unit A

Matching

1.	c	**8.**	m
2.	h	**9.**	l
3.	e	**10.**	d
4.	k	**11.**	j
5.	n	**12.**	g
6.	f	**13.**	i
7.	a	**14.**	b

Outline

1.	B	**12.**	H
2.	C	**13.**	K
3.	F	**14.**	R
4.	I	**15.**	S
5.	L	**16.**	T
6.	M	**17.**	U
7.	N	**18.**	V
8.	O	**19.**	A
9.	P	**20.**	G
10.	D	**21.**	J
11.	E	**22.**	Q

Multiple Choice

1.	c	**12.**	b
2.	d	**13.**	d
3.	a	**14.**	a
4.	c	**15.**	d
5.	c	**16.**	a
6.	a	**17.**	d
7.	a	**18.**	a
8.	c	**19.**	d
9.	d	**20.**	c
10.	b	**21.**	a
11.	c	**22.**	b

Crossword

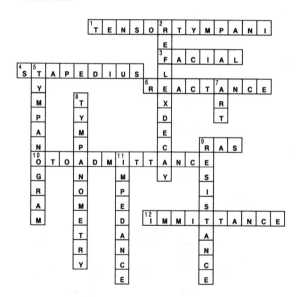

Activity

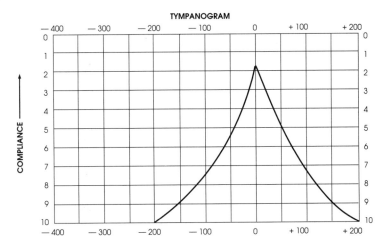

FIGURE 5A-5.   Type A.

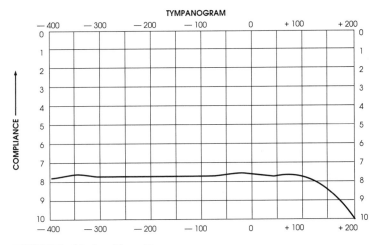

FIGURE 5A-6.   Type B.

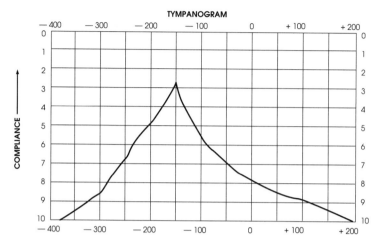

FIGURE 5A-7.   Type C.

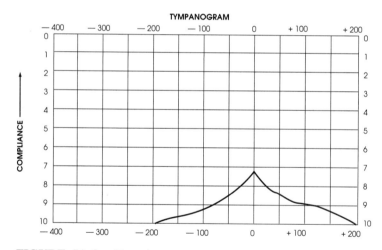

FIGURE 5A-8.   Type A$_S$.

UNIT B: ELECTROPHYSIOLOGICAL TESTS OF HEARING

Background

The dream of any audiologist would be to find a test that accurately reveals the hearing sensitivity of noncooperative patients. Such patients include infants and small children, persons who are mentally challenged, and pseudohypacusic individuals. Because the body responds to sound through both the central and autonomic nervous systems, the challenge has been to find the modality to monitor and a means of doing it accurately. Measurements in response to sound have been made to changes in heart rate, skin resistance, respiration, pupil size, and brain-wave activity. Once popular as a diagnostic test is the electrodermal response, which is largely in disuse because of the great potential for misinterpretation and the necessity of presenting uncomfortable and sometimes painful electric shocks as conditioning stimuli. Monitoring of electrical responses in the brain on an electroencephalograph was made difficult by the fact that the electrical response itself is of significantly smaller amplitude than the ongoing electrical activity of a living brain. The development of averaging computers allows the presentation of numbers of stimuli so that the background activity can be averaged to near zero amplitude while the series of waves that signify responses at different points following stimulus introduction are increased in amplitude. All this serves to improve the signal-to-noise ratio. Responses that are observed with a latency (time after stimulus onset) greater than 50 milliseconds are thought to occur in the auditory cortex. Results with cortical evoked responses were hopeful at first but led to disappointment. Of greatest interest today is the auditory brain-stem response, which is represented by seven small wavelets in the first 10 milliseconds after click stimulation. The auditory brainstem response currently is used not only as a test of hearing but also to help in determination of the site of auditory lesion. Promising research is ongoing with the middle latency response.

Objectives

1. You should know and understand the terms in the matching exercise.
2. You should be able to fill in the outline, selecting items from the list provided.
3. You should be able to answer the multiple-choice questions on electrophysiological tests.
4. You should be able to complete the crossword puzzle.

Matching

Match the term from the column on the right with its definition.

Definition

1. ___ Evoked potentials that appear 10 to 50 msec after signal onset (abbr.)

2. ___ Evoked potentials that appear 75 msec after signal onset with a large wave at a latency of 300 msec (abbr.)

3. ___ The third electrode used in auditory evoked potential testing that prevents the body from acting as an antenna

4. ___ The electrode used in auditory evoked potential testing that is unaffected by electrical activity in the brain

5. ___ Evoked potentials that appear within the first 10 msec after signal onset (abbr.)

6. ___ Evoked potentials that occur almost immediately after signal onset

7. ___ A graph drawn as a function of the delay in appearance of wave V versus the intensity required to produce the wave

8. ___ Evoked potentials that appear about 100 msec after signal onset

Term

a. ABR

b. Auditory event related

c. AMLR

d. ECochG

e. Ground

f. LER

g. Latency-intensity

h. Reference

Outline

Electrophysiological Tests

ABR

Stimulus

1. _____

Equipment

2. _____

3. _____

Select From

A. Averaging computer

B. Clicks or tone bursts

C. Promontory electrodes and amplifier

D. Pure tone

E. Scalp electrodes and amplifier

F. 1–10 msec

G. 50–300 msec

Response Latency

4. _____

ECochG

Stimulus

5. _____

Equipment

6. _____

7. _____

Response Latency

8. _____

LER

Stimulus

9. _____

Equipment

10. _____

11. _____

Response Latency

12. _____

Multiple Choice

1. Auditory brain-stem response audiometry views responses to sounds that occur
   a. immediately after the stimulus
   b. 350 msec after the stimulus
   c. visually
   d. never

2. One very important device for performing auditory evoked response audiometry is a
   a. psychogalvanometer
   b. Wheatstone bridge
   c. averaging computer
   d. inductorium

3. During electrocochleography, the target electrode is not placed on the
   a. round window
   b. promontory
   c. external auditory canal
   d. mastoid process

4. During ABR the most reliable wave in normal hearing adults is number
   a. III
   b. IV
   c. V
   d. VI

5. Middle latency responses are those that occur ___ msec after the presentation of the signal
   a. 0–10
   b. 10–50
   c. 50–100
   d. 100–300

6. The usual stimulus for ABR is a
   a. click
   b. pure tone
   c. narrow-band noise
   d. wideband noise

7. During ABR the average electrical response is
   a. 1–5 millivolts
   b. 1–5 microvolts
   c. 1–5 volts
   d. none of the above

8. ECochG has an advantage over ABR in that
   a. bone conduction can be done without masking
   b. the test is less involved
   c. the test takes less time
   d. subjects need not be anesthetized

9. ABR results are an indication of
   a. neural integrity
   b. hearing loss in the 250 to 500 Hz range
   c. hearing loss in the 6000 to 8000 Hz range
   d. cortical function

10. The event-related potential is also called the
    a. ABR
    b. P300
    c. AMLR
    d. ECochG

11. Otoacoustic emissions occurring in the absence of external stimulation are called
    a. SOAE
    b. TEOAE
    c. EOAE
    d. DPOAE

12. Two primary tones are required when measuring
    a. SOAE
    b. TEOAE
    c. EOAE
    d. DPOAE

13. Otoacoustic emissions are usually absent in
    a. cochlear hearing loss
    b. conductive hearing loss
    c. VIIIth nerve hearing loss
    d. a & b

14. A patient with a moderate hearing loss and present evoked otoacoustic emissions probably has a
    a. cochlear lesion
    b. conductive loss
    c. mixed loss
    d. VIIIth nerve loss

Crossword

Across

2. Auditory evoked potentials that occur 10 to 50 msec after stimulus
3. The electrode used in testing auditory evoked potentials that is unaffected by brain activity
5. A sound, originating in the cochlea, that can abe detected in the outer ear (abbr.)
7. A graph showing the delay in appearance of wave V (2 words)
11. An echo produced by the cochlea (abbr.)

Down

1. The electrode used to prevent reception of extraneous electrical signals
4. The auditory evoked potential that shows its largest wave at 300 msec latency (2 words)
6. Auditory evoked potentials that occur after a latency of more than 100 msec (abbr.)
8. Auditory evoked potentials that occur within the first 10 msec after stimulation (abbr.)
9. A sound that can be detected in the outer ear that requires no external stimulation (abbr.)
10. An otoacoustic emission evoked by transient stimuli (abbr.)
12. Electrical response to a sound that occurs almost immediately after stimulus onset (abbr.)

Crossword

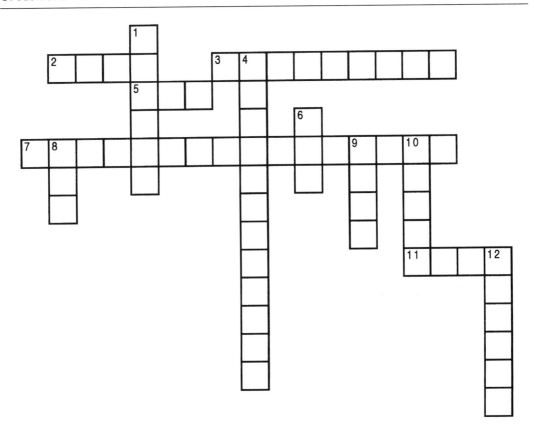

Answers—Unit B

Matching

1.	c	**5.**	a
2.	b	**6.**	d
3.	e	**7.**	g
4.	h	**8.**	f

Outline

1.	B	**7.**	C
2.	A	**8.**	F
3.	E	**9.**	D
4.	F	**10.**	A
5.	B	**11.**	E
6.	A	**12.**	G

Multiple Choice

1.	a	**8.**	a
2.	c	**9.**	a
3.	d	**10.**	b
4.	c	**11.**	a
5.	b	**12.**	b
6.	a	**13.**	d
7.	b	**14.**	d

Crossword

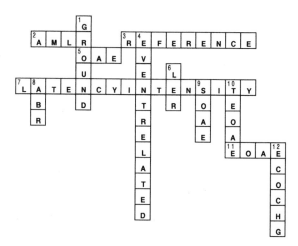

UNIT C: BEHAVIORAL TESTS FOR SITE OF LESION

Background

Through the years a number of special tests have been developed based on different psychoacoustic phenomena. Lesions in various areas of the hearing system alter the responses on some of these tests. One phenomenon, loudness recruitment (the large increase in loudness with relatively small increases in intensity seen in patients with cochlear lesions), has led to the development of the Alternate Binaural Loudness Balance (ABLB) test. As an offshoot of the difference limen for intensity, the Short Increment Sensitivity Index (SISI) emerged as a means of determining cochlear lesions and was later modified to test for retrocochlear sites. Studies examining the speed with which a continuous tone fades from audibility depending on auditory pathology resulted in a number of different tone decay tests. By using the method of adjustment with the patient in control of the intensity of puretone signals, Békésy (automatic) audiometry results in tracking behavior that may be different for continuous versus automatically pulsed tones. Although none of these tests is consistently accurate, when they are used together as a battery, the result is often a constellation that helps to identify the locus of disorder within the auditory system.

Objectives

1. You should know and understand the terms in the matching exercise.
2. You should be able to fill in the outline, selecting items from the list provided.
3. You should understand the principles underlying the ABLB test, the equipment required, and how the test is performed.
4. You should understand the principles underlying the SISI test, the equipment required, and how the test is performed.
5. You should understand the principles underlying the tone decay test, the equipment required, and how the test is performed.
6. You should understand the principles underlying Békésy audiometry, the equipment required, and how the test is performed.
7. You should be able to list the kinds of results on each of the above tests that theoretically would be expected from patients with conductive, cochlear, and retrocochlear lesions.
8. You should be able to complete the activities in this unit.
9. You should be able to answer the multiple-choice questions and understand the purposes and uses of behavioral tests for site of auditory lesion.
10. You should be able to complete the crossword puzzle.

Matching

Match the term or abbreviation from the column on the right with its definition.

Definition

1. ___ A condition in which an intense sound is almost as loud to an impaired ear as it is to a normal ear

2. ___ A tone decay test carried out near the limits of an audiometer

3. ___ A test of perstimulatory adaptation

4. ___ Comparison of a comfortable level for pulsed and continuous tones, carried out on an automatic audiometer

5. ___ A test of loudness recruitment requiring the patient to have one normal and one hearing impaired ear

6. ___ The less-than-normal growth of loudness of a signal as intensity is increased

7. ___ A plot for illustrating results on an ABLB or AMLB test

8. ___ A test to determine whether a patient can detect a change in the loudness of a tone when the intensity is increased by 1 dB

9. ___ A condition in which an intense sound is louder in an impaired ear than it is in a normal ear at the same intensity

10. ___ A procedure using automatic audiometry that compares a patient's thresholds for pulsed and continuous tones

11. ___ Perstimulatory adaptation to a pure tone

12. ___ The score (in percentage) on a test of word recognition

13. ___ The ability of a listener to barely detect small changes in intensity as changes in loudness

Term

a. ABLB

b. AMLB

c. Békésy audiometry

d. BCL

e. Decruitment

f. DLI

g. Hyperrecruitment

h. Laddergram

i. Partial

j. Recruitment

k. SISI

l. STAT

m. Tone decay

n. TDT

o. Word-recognition score

Definition

14. ___ A relatively large increase in loudness resulting from a small increase in intensity

15. ___ A test of loudness recruitment requiring the patient to have normal and impaired hearing at two frequencies in the same ear

Outline

Behavioral Tests

ABLB

Test for

1. _____

Type of Loss

2. _____

Results

3. _____

4. _____

5. _____

6. _____

7. _____

Equipment

8. _____

SISI

Test for

9. _____

Type of Loss

10. _____

11. _____

Select From

A. Audiometer and stopwatch

B. Békésy audiometer

C. Bilateral loss

D. Decruitment—retrocochlear

E. Detect 1–dB increments

F. Equal loudness in both ears at the same intensity

G. Hyperrecruitment—cochlear

H. No recruitment—conductive or retrocochlear

I. Partial recruitment—cochlear

J. Recruitment—cochlear

K. Separation of pulsed and continuous threshold tracings

L. SISI adapter

M. Tone fades to inaudibility

N. Tone loses musical quality

O. Type I—no decay—normal or conductive

P. Type I—no separation between pulsed and continuous—conductive

Q. Type II—slight decay—cochlear

R. Type II—continuous worse than pulsed in high frequencies—cochlear

Behavioral Tests

Results

12. _____

13. _____

14. _____

Equipment

15. _____

Tone Decay

Test for

16. _____

17. _____

Type of Loss

18. _____

19. _____

Results

20. _____

21. _____

22. _____

Equipment

23. _____

Békésy Audiometry

Test For

24. _____

Type of Loss

25. _____

26. _____

Select From

S. Type III—marked decay—retrocochlear

T. Type III—continuous much worse than pulsed at all frequencies—retrocochlear

U. Type IV—continuous slightly worse than pulsed at all frequencies—possible retrocochlear

V. Type V—pulsed worse than continuous—pseudohypacusis

W. Two channel audiometer

X. Unilateral loss

Y. 0–25 percent—noncochlear

Z. 30–70 percent indeterminable

AA. 75–100 percent—cochlear

Results

27. _____

28. _____

29. _____

30. _____

31. _____

Equipment

32. _____

Activities

ABLB

Six laddergrams are shown in Figure 5C-1. The first is a model showing normal hearing in both ears. The other five show a 40-dB hearing loss in the right ear and normal hearing in the left ear. Show the theoretical levels in the left ear that are equal in loudness to 60 and 80 dB in the right ear for each of the following conditions: (B) no recruitment, (C) complete recruitment, (D) partial recruitment, (E) hyperrecruitment, and (F) decruitment. Compare your laddergrams to the correct ones (Figure 5C-3) at the end of this unit.

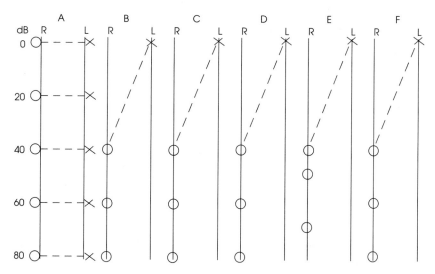

FIGURE 5C-1. Six laddergrams.

Békésy Audiometry

Five Békésy tracings are shown in Figure 5C-2 (P = pulsed tone; C= continuous tone). Put the numbered type in the indicated place and write in the letter that corresponds to the suggested site of lesion: (A) conductive loss, (B) cochlear loss, (C) retrocochlear loss, and (D) pseudohypacusis.

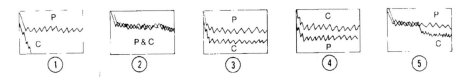

FIGURE 5C-2.   Five Békésy tracings.

   1. Type _____

       Site _____

   2. Type _____

       Site _____

   3. Type _____

       Site _____

   4. Type _____

       Site _____

   5. Type _____

       Site _____

Multiple Choice

   1. A SISI score of 50 percent suggests
      a. cochlear lesion
      b. retrocochlear lesion
      c. conductive lesion
      d. unknown

2. When recruitment is present
- **a.** loudness grows so rapidly that a tone may be as loud in the impaired ear as it is in the normal ear at the same SPL
- **b.** loudness grows more slowly in the impaired ear than it does in a normal ear
- **c.** loudness grows more quickly than normal in the impaired ear but without complete recruitment
- **d.** there is no growth of loudness in the impaired ear

3. Normal-hearing individuals would be expected to get 100 percent SISI scores at ___ dB HL
- **a.** 10
- **b.** 20
- **c.** 40
- **d.** 80

4. The presence of loudness recruitment suggests
- **a.** conductive hearing loss
- **b.** normal hearing
- **c.** cochlear hearing loss
- **d.** retrocochlear loss

5. A patient has normal hearing in both ears but an VIIIth nerve lesion on the left side. SISI scores using 1 dB increments at 90 dB HL would probably be
- **a.** left 0 percent, right 0 percent
- **b.** left 100 percent, right 100 percent
- **c.** left 0 percent, right 100 percent
- **d.** left 100 percent, right 0 percent

6. In addition to threshold tracing, Békésy audiometry may be useful diagnostically in tracking
- **a.** MCL
- **b.** SDS
- **c.** SRT
- **d.** 50 dB SL

7. Given a right cortical lesion, one would expect
- **a.** recruitment in the right ear
- **b.** recruitment in the left ear
- **c.** decruitment in the right ear
- **d.** decruitment in the left ear

8. During Békésy audiometry, a patient tracks the continuous tone at 50 dB and the interrupted tone at 70 dB. This would suggest
- **a.** conductive loss
- **b.** cochlear loss
- **c.** VIIIth nerve loss
- **d.** none of the above

9. Type II Békésy tracings are characterized by
   a. continuous poorer than pulsed at 1000 Hz and above
   b. continuous poorer than pulsed at 250 Hz and above
   c. continuous poorer than pulsed through the frequency range
   d. continuous and pulsed superimposed through the frequency range

10. The tone decay test that requires the patient to report a change in the quality of the tone is attributed to
    a. Green
    b. Olsen and Noffsinger
    c. Carhart
    d. Rosenberg

11. The tone decay test that is begun at 20 dB above the patient's threshold is attributed to
    a. Green
    b. Olsen and Noffsinger
    c. Carhart
    d. Rosenberg

12. The first tone decay test that could be completed in one minute per frequency is attributed to
    a. Green
    b. Olsen and Noffsinger
    c. Carhart
    d. Rosenberg

13. The high-intensity tone decay test is called
    a. STOP
    b. STAT
    c. START
    d. none of the above

14. In Békésy audiometry, separation between pulsed and continuous tracings is enhanced by
    a. sweeping from 100 to 10,000 Hz
    b. sweeping from 10,000 to 100 Hz
    c. using fixed frequency tracings
    d. not sweeping

15. To use the ABLB test the patient must have
    a. normal hearing in one ear and a hearing loss in the other ear
    b. normal hearing at one frequency in one ear and a hearing loss at a different frequency in the other ear
    c. normal hearing at one frequency and a hearing loss at a different frequency in the same ear
    d. hearing loss at all frequencies in both ears

16. Diagnosis of site of lesion is best accomplished by interactions among or between
   a. SISI and Békésy
   b. ABLB and TDT
   c. SISI, ABLB, and TDT
   d. Békésy, SISI, TDT, and ABLB

17. The site-of-lesion test considered to have the greatest sensitivity is
   a. ABLB
   b. ABR
   c. SISI
   d. tone decay

Crossword

Across

2. A test for abnormal loudness growth on patients with unilateral hearing loss (abbr.)
7. Extremely rapid growth of loudness with respect to intensity
8. A test for loudness growth that compares two frequencies in the same ear (abbr.)
10. Abnormal growth of loudness with respect to intensity
12. Perstimulatory adaptation (2 words)
14. A test for perstimulatory adaptation (abbr.)

Down

1. A means of plotting the results of recruitment tests
3. Abnormally slow growth of loudness with respect to intensity
4. Patient's tracking of levels of comfortable loudness using automatic audiometry (abbr.)
5. A test for detection of small changes in intensity (acronym)
6. A test for perstimulatory adaptation performed at high intensities (acronym)
9. Automatic audiometry
11. The result on a test of loudness growth that shows nearly complete
13. The ability to barely detect changes in the loudness of a signal (abbr.)

Crossword

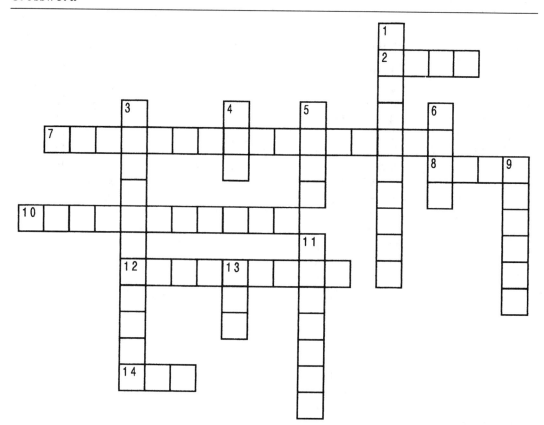

Answers—Unit C

Matching

1.	I	**9.**	g
2.	l	**10.**	c
3.	n	**11.**	m
4.	d	**12.**	o
5.	a	**13.**	f
6.	e	**14.**	j
7.	h	**15.**	b
8.	k		

Outline

1.	F	**17.**	N
2.	X	**18.**	C
3.	D	**19.**	X
4.	G	**20.**	O
5.	H	**21.**	Q
6.	I	**22.**	S
7.	J	**23.**	A
8.	W	**24.**	K
9.	E	**25.**	C
10.	C	**26.**	X
11.	X	**27.**	P
12.	Y	**28.**	R
13.	Z	**29.**	T
14.	AA	**30.**	U
15.	L	**31.**	V
16.	M	**32.**	B

Activities

Békésy Audiometry

Type		Site
1.	III	C
2.	I	A
3.	IV	C
4.	V	D
5.	II	B

Multiple Choice

1.	d	**10.**	a
2.	a	**11.**	b
3.	d	**12.**	d
4.	c	**13.**	b
5.	c	**14.**	b
6.	a	**15.**	a
7.	d	**16.**	d
8.	d	**17.**	b
9.	a		

Crossword

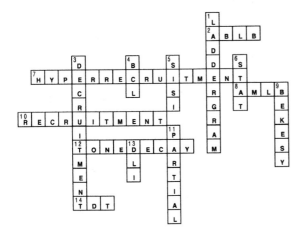

ABLB

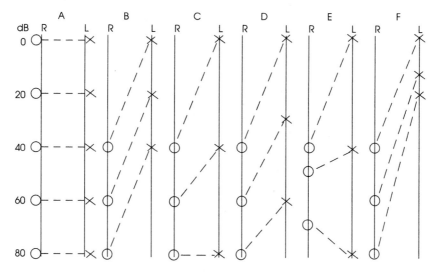

FIGURE 5C-3. Correct laddergrams.

Chapter 6

The Outer Ear

Background

The outer ear is the most visible part of the auditory system and is made up primarily of a funnel-like appendage, a resonating tube, and a vibrating membrane. Its function is to gather sound waves from the environment and allow them to propagate to the eardrum membrane. Any material that blocks the passageway can cause a conductive hearing loss.

Objectives

1. You should know and understand the terms in the matching exercise.
2. You should be able to fill in the outline, selecting items from the list provided.
3. You should be able to label parts of the outer ear and tympanic membrane in Figures 6-1, 6-2, and 6-3.
4. You should be able to answer the multiple-choice questions and understand the anatomy and physiology of the outer ear, as well as the causes of disorders that produce conductive hearing loss.
5. You should be able to complete the crossword puzzle.

Matching

Match the term from the column on the right with its definition.

Definition	*Term*
1. E Earwax	a. Agenesis
2. J A special light designed for looking into the ear	b. Anotia
	c. Atresia
3. B Absence of the pinna	d. Auricle
4. M The same as pars flaccida	e. Cerumen
5. G Inflammation of the external ear	f. External auditory canal
6. K The tense portion of the tympanic membrane, making up its largest area and consisting of three layers	g. External otitis
	h. Myringoplasty
7. D The appendage of the external ear consisting of cartilage	i. Otalgia
	j. Otoscope
8. H Surgery to repair the tympanic membrane	k. Pars flaccida
9. L The point of the tympanic membrane that is approximately in the center	l. Pars tensa
	m. Shrapnell's membrane
10. C Closure of a body orifice that is normally open	n. Tympanic membrane
	o. Umbo
11. M The flabby portion of the tympanic membrane found near the top	
12. N The membrane that vibrates to allow sound to enter the middle ear from the outer ear	
13. I Ear pain	
14. E The channel that conducts sound from the auricle to the tympanic membrane	
15. A Failure of a portion of the anatomy to develop	

Outline

The Outer Ear

Anatomy

1. _____

2. _____

3. _____

4. _____

Disorders

5. _____

6. _____

7. _____

8. _____

9. _____

10. _____

Surgical Treatment

11. _____

12. _____

Select Fr...

A. Atresia

B. Bony ex...

C. Cartilagi... ...ternal ear canal

D. Foreign bodies

E. Infections

F. Myringoplasty

G. Perforations

H. Pinna

I. Tympanic membrane

J. Tympanoplasty

K. Tumors

L. Wax

Label the parts of the pinna, outer ear, and tympanic membrane in the figures that follow. Select the terms from the lists provided.

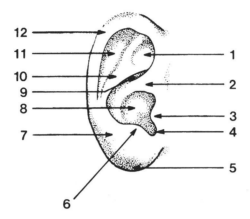

FIGURE 6-1.   The pinna (auricle).

Label

1. _____
2. _____
3. _____
4. _____
5. _____

Term

A. Auricle (pinna)
B. Bony external auditory canal
C. Cartilaginous external auditory canal
D. Mastoid air cells
E. Tympanic membrane

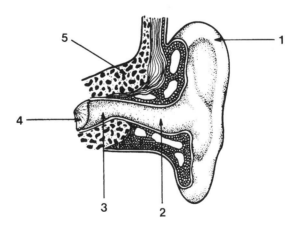

FIGURE 6-2.   The Outer Ear

Label

1. _____
2. _____
3. _____
4. _____
5. _____
6. _____
7. _____
8. _____
9. _____
10. _____
11. _____
12. _____

Term

A. Antihelix
B. Antitragus
C. Cavum concha
D. Crus of helix
E. Cymba concha
F. Helix
G. Intertragal notch
H. Lobe
I. Scaphoid fossa
J. Tragus
K. Triangular fossa

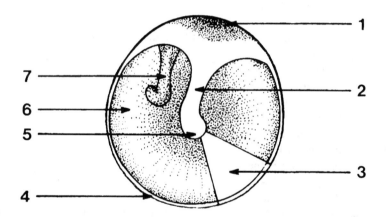

FIGURE 6-3.   The tympanic membrane.

Label

1. _____
2. _____
3. _____
4. _____
5. _____
6. _____
7. _____

Term

A. Annular ligament
B. Cone of light
C. Long process of incus
D. Manubrium of malleus
E. Pars flaccida
F. Pars tensa
G. Umbo

Multiple Choice

1. Cerumen is produced in the
   a. entire external auditory canal
   b. cartilaginous external auditory canal
   c. osseous external auditory canal
   d. temporomandibular joint
2. Congenital absence of the external auditory canal is called
   a. microtia
   b. stenosis
   c. minutia
   d. atresia
3. The portion of the tympanic membrane in which the malleus is embedded is the
   a. umbo
   b. annulus
   c. cone of light
   d. pars tensa
4. A large central perforation of the tympanic membrane theoretically results in hearing that is
   a. normal
   b. slightly to moderately impaired
   c. severely impaired
   d. profoundly impaired
5. A term for a bacterial infection of the outer ear is
   a. otomycosis
   b. cerumen in the lumen
   c. otitis media
   d. external otitis
6. The portion of the tympanic membrane that does not contain the fibrocartilaginous layer is the
   a. umbo
   b. pars tensa
   c. pars flaccida
   d. annulus
7. In air-conduction audiometry, a loss of the pinna results in
   a. no hearing loss
   b. mild sensorineural hearing loss
   c. mild conductive hearing loss
   d. mild mixed hearing loss
8. The point of maximum retraction of the tympanic membrane is the
   a. annulus
   b. concha
   c. umbo
   d. pars flaccida

9. The resonant frequency of the external auditory canal is
   a. 500–2000 Hz
   b. 3000–5000 Hz
   c. 8000–10,000 Hz
   d. 10,000–12,000 Hz
10. The innermost layer of the tympanic membrane (on the middle-ear side) is covered with
    a. epidermis
    b. fibrous material
    c. mucous membrane
    d. muscle
11. The cone of light of the tympanic membrane is
    a. superior-anterior
    b. superior-posterior
    c. inferior-anterior
    d. inferior-posterior
12. Narrowing of the external auditory canal is called
    a. atresia
    b. stenosis
    c. otitis
    d. otomycosis

Crossword

Across

2. An abnormally small pinna
4. Absence of the pinna
7. The cartilaginous appendage at the external ear
8. The middle primary embryonic germ layer
9. The outermost primary embryonic germ layer
10. Plastic surgery on the auricle
11. Infection of the outer ear (2 words)
15. A specially designed light for looking into the external ear
16. The ring of cartilage around the tympanic membrane
18. The syndrome causing ear pain because of jaw misalignment (abbr.)
19. Surgery to repair the tympanic membrane

Down

1. The largest part of the tympanic membrane containing three tissue layers (2 words)
2. Inflammation of the tympanic membrane
3. The external channel that allows sound to reach the eardrum membrane (2 words)
5. Earwax
6. Pain in the ear
10. The flabby portion at the top of the tympanic membrane that is made up of two layers (2 words)
11. The innermost primary embryonic germ layer
12. The membrane often called the eardrum
13. Closure of a normally open orifice, such as the external auditory canal
14. Plastic surgery on the ear
17. A point at the approximate center of the eardrum membrane

Crossword

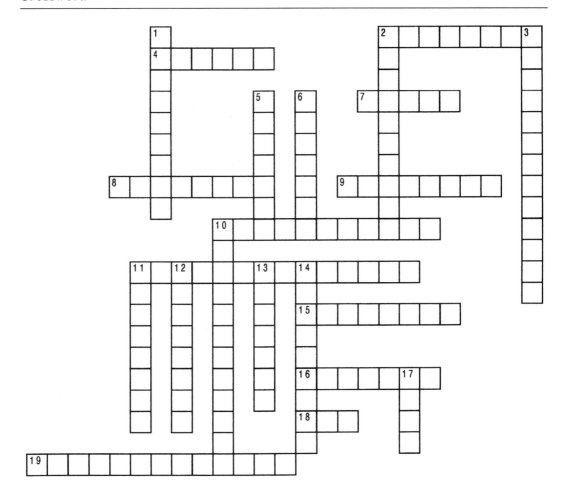

Answers

Matching

1.	e	9.	o
2.	j	10.	c
3.	b	11.	k
4.	m	12.	n
5.	f	13.	i
6.	l	14.	f
7.	d	15.	a

Activities

Pinna

1.	K	7.	F
2.	D	8.	C
3.	J	9.	E
4.	G	10.	A
5.	H	11.	I
6.	B	12.	F

Outer Ear

1.	A
2.	C
3.	B
4.	E
5.	D

Tympanic Membrane

1.	E
2.	D
3.	B
4.	A
5.	G
6.	F
7.	C

Multiple Choice

1.	b	7.	a
2.	d	8.	c
3.	d	9.	b
4.	b	10.	c
5.	d	11.	c
6.	c	12.	b

Crossword

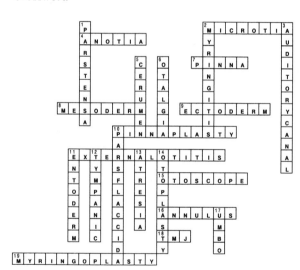

C h a p t e r 7

The Middle Ear

Background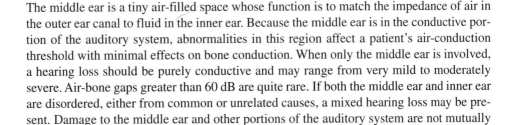

The middle ear is a tiny air-filled space whose function is to match the impedance of air in the outer ear canal to fluid in the inner ear. Because the middle ear is in the conductive portion of the auditory system, abnormalities in this region affect a patient's air-conduction threshold with minimal effects on bone conduction. When only the middle ear is involved, a hearing loss should be purely conductive and may range from very mild to moderately severe. Air-bone gaps greater than 60 dB are quite rare. If both the middle ear and inner ear are disordered, either from common or unrelated causes, a mixed hearing loss may be present. Damage to the middle ear and other portions of the auditory system are not mutually exclusive. Dysfunction of the middle ear may result from disease, trauma, or hereditary conditions.

Objectives

1. You should know and understand the terms in the matching exercise.
2. You should be able to fill in the outline, selecting items from the list provided.
3. You should be able to label the different parts of the middle ear shown in Figure 7-1.
4. You should be able to answer the multiple-choice questions and understand the anatomy and physiology of the middle ear as well as the causes of disorders that produce conductive hearing loss.
5. You should be able to complete the crossword puzzle.

Matching

Match the term from the column on the right with its definition.

Definition

1. ___ The largest of the ossicles, which is attached to the tympanic membrane

2. ___ An operation to reverse hearing loss caused by otosclerosis, carried out by breaking the footplate of the stapes free

3. ___ An artifact in bone conduction in patients with otosclerosis

4. ___ A surgical procedure to restore the middle-ear function

5. ___ The VIIth cranial nerve

6. ___ The second bone in the ossicular chain that connects the malleus to the stapes

7. ___ The chain of three tiny bones in the middle ear

8. ___ Sterile fluid accumulation in the middle ear

9. ___ An operation to remove infection from the mastoid

10. ___ A space in the superior portion of the middle-ear space

11. ___ The Vth cranial nerve

12. ___ A small muscle that can impede movement of the malleus

13. ___ Inflammation of the mastoid

14. ___ An operation designed to improve hearing loss caused by otosclerosis by removing the stapes and replacing it with a prosthesis

15. ___ The attic of the middle-ear space

16. ___ The moist lining of the middle-ear space

17. ___ Infection of the middle ear

18. ___ In anatomy, a leg, as of the stapes

Term

a. Aditus
b. Carhart notch
c. Cholesteatoma
d. Crus
e. Epitympanic recess
f. Eustachian tube
g. Facial nerve
h. Fenestration
i. Incus
j. Malleus
k. Mastoidectomy
l. Mastoiditis
m. Mucous membrane
n. Myringotomy
o. Ossicles
p. Otitis media
q. Otosclerosis
r. Oval window
s. Round window
t. Serous effusion
u. Stapedectomy
v. Stapedius muscle
w. Stapes
x. Stapes mobilization
y. Tensor tympani muscle
z. Trigeminal nerve
aa. Tympanoplasty
ab. Tympanosclerosis

19. ___ Formation of spongy bone that may affect the normal movement of the stapes

20. ___ Incision into the tympanic membrane, usually to remove fluid

21. ___ A membrane separating the middle ear from the inner ear

22. ___ A channel connecting the middle ear to the nasopharynx

23. ___ Calcium formations in the middle ear, often caused by infection

24. ___ The smallest of the ossicles, which stands in the oval window

25. ___ An older operation to correct hearing loss from otosclerosis

26. ___ A membrane, supporting the footplate of the stapes, that separates the middle ear from the inner ear

27. ___ A small muscle, connected to the stapes, that impedes movement of the ossicles when it is contracted

28. ___ A collection of fats and other debris in the middle ear, usually caused by infection

Outline

The Middle Ear

Anatomy

1. _____

2. _____

3. _____

4. _____

5. _____

6. _____

7. _____

Select From

A. Aditus ad antrum
B. Congenital abnormalities
C. Epitympanic recess
D. Eustachian tube
E. Fenestration
F. Fractures
G. Incus
H. Malleus
I. Mastoidectomy
J. Middle ear space
K. Myringotomy

The Middle Ear

Bones

8. _____

9. _____

10. _____

Muscles

11. _____

12. _____

13. _____

Disorders

14. _____

15. _____

16. _____

17. _____

18. _____

Surgical Treatment

19. _____

20. _____

21. _____

22. _____

23. _____

24. _____

Select From

L. Otitis media
M. Otosclerosis
N. Oval window
O. Round window
P. Serous effusion
Q. Stapedectomy
R. Stapes
S. Stapes mobilization
T. Stapedius
U. Tensor tympani
V. Tympanic membrane
W. Tympanoplasty
X. Tympanosclerosis

Activity

Select the terms from the list provided and label the parts of the middle ear in the figure below.

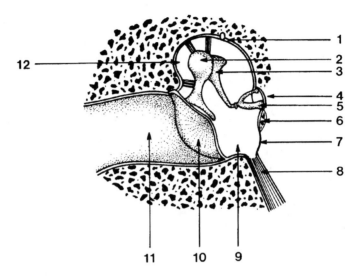

FIGURE 7.1   The middle ear.

Label

1. _____
2. _____
3. _____
4. _____
5. _____
6. _____
7. _____

Bones

8. _____

9. _____
10. _____

Muscles

11. _____
12. _____

Term

A. Aditus ad antrum
B. Epitympanic recess
C. Eustachian tube
D. External auditory canal
E. Incus
F. Malleus
G. Middle-ear space
H. Oval window
I. Promontory
J. Round window
K. Stapes
L. Tympanic membrane

Multiple Choice

1. The chain of bones in the middle ear is called the
   a. malleus
   b. incus
   c. stapes
   d. ossicles

2. Stapedectomy has replaced stapes mobilization because
   a. there is less possibility of refixation
   b. the potential air-bone gap is small
   c. the operation is tolerated better
   d. it is less dangerous to perform

3. The general classification of surgical procedures for repairing damage of middle ear structures is
   a. tympanoplasty
   b. stapedialplasty
   c. rhinoplasty
   d. otoplasty

4. A pseudotumor in the middle ear composed of skin and fatty tissue is called
   a. otitis externa
   b. otosclerosis
   c. otitis media
   d. cholesteatoma

5. Which of the following is *not* a usual treatment for serous effusion?
   a. pressure-equalizing tubes
   b. mastoidectomy
   c. myringotomy
   d. decongestant medication

6. Pressure-equalizing tubes are designed to function primarily as an artificial
   a. ear canal
   b. mastoid
   c. eustachian tube
   d. hairpiece

7. The most popular surgical treatment for otosclerosis is
   a. fenestration
   b. tympanoplasty
   c. stapedectomy
   d. stapes mobilization

8. The manubrium is part of the
   a. malleus
   b. incus
   c. stapes
   d. eustachian tube

9. The eustachian tube connects the middle ear with the
   a. outer ear
   b. inner ear
   c. nasopharynx
   d. nose
10. Nonbacterial otitis media usually results from
    a. a blocked eustachian tube
    b. nasopharyngitis
    c. otitis media
    d. otosclerosis
11. Otosclerosis is
    a. equally common in men and women
    b. more common in men
    c. more common in women
    d. most common in children
12. Fluid in the middle-ear space may result from
    a. a blocked eustachian tube
    b. infection entering the middle ear via the eustachian tube
    c. infection entering the middle ear via the bloodstream
    d. all of the above
13. Hearing speech better in a noisy place than in a quiet place is a symptom of
    a. normal hearing
    b. conductive hearing loss
    c. sensorineural hearing loss
    d. none of the above
14. The Carhart notch is usually associated with
    a. otosclerosis
    b. bacterial otitis media
    c. serous effusion
    d. a blocked eustachian tube
15. Given a moderate conductive hearing loss in the right ear and normal hearing in the left ear, otoacoustic emissions are expected to be
    a. absent in both ear
    b. present in both ears
    c. present in the right ear, absent in the left ear
    d. present in the left ear, absent in the right ear

Crossword

Across

2. Infection of the mastoid bone
4. The tube that connects the middle ear with the nasopharnyx
5. An older operation to improve hearing loss caused by otosclerosis
7. a pseudotumor found in the middle ear
15. The window separating the middle ear from the inner ear that is below the promontory
16. In anatomy a "leg," such as on the stapes
17. The muscle that attaches to the malleus
18. The chain of three tiny bones in each middle ear

Down

1. An artifact in bone conduction caused by otosclerosis (2 words)
3. The middlemost bone of the ossicular chain, sometimes called the anvil
6. The largest and first of the middle-ear bones, sometimes called the hammer
8. Formation of a new bone growth that can immobilize the stapes
9. Third and smallest of the middle-ear bones, sometimes called the stirrup
10. The space at the top of the middle ear
11. The window separating the middle ear from the inner ear that supports the stapes
12. Incision into the tympanic membrane
13. Infection of the middle-ear space (2 words)
14. The VIIth cranial nerve

Crossword

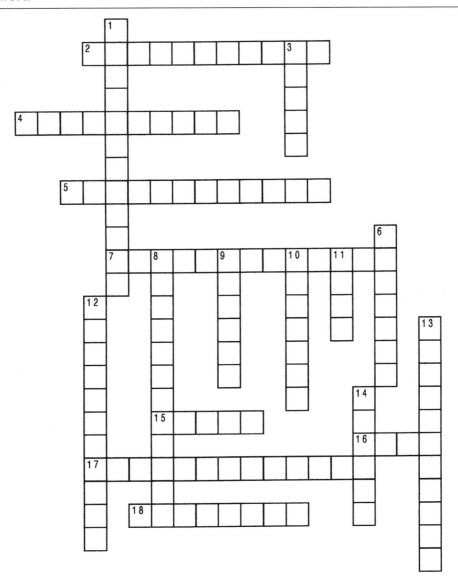

Answers To Chapter 7

Matching

1. j	**11.** z	**21.** s
2. x	**12.** y	**22.** f
3. b	**13.** l	**23.** ab
4. aa	**14.** u	**24.** w
5. g	**15.** e	**25.** h
6. i	**16.** m	**26.** r
7. o	**17.** p	**27.** v
8. t	**18.** d	**28.** c
9. k	**19.** q	
10. a	**20.** n	

Outline

1. A	**13.** B
2. C	**14.** F
3. D	**15.** L
4. J	**16.** M
5. N	**17.** P
6. O	**18.** X
7. V	**19.** E
8. G	**20.** I
9. H	**21.** K
10. R	**22.** Q
11. T	**23.** S
12. U	**24.** W

Activity

1. A	**7.** J
2. F	**8.** C
3. E	**9.** G
4. H	**10.** L
5. K	**11.** D
6. I	**12.** B

Multiple Choice

1. d	**9.** c
2. a	**10.** a
3. a	**11.** c
4. d	**12.** d
5. b	**13.** b
6. c	**14.** a
7. c	**15.** d
8. a	

Crossword

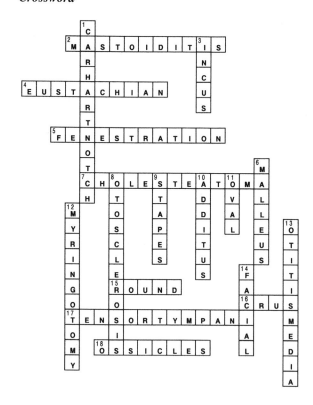

Chapter 8

The Inner Ear

UNIT A: STRUCTURE, FUNCTION, AND DISORDERS

Background

The inner ear is often called a *labyrinth*, which is Greek for a series of winding passages. Although extremely tiny, it is a myriad of hydromechanical and neuroelectric activity. Through its vestibular apparatus the inner ear provides the brain with the sensation of the head's position and motion in space. Through the cochlea the inner ear converts the mechanical acoustical vibrations of the middle ear into a form of energy, which the brain ultimately perceives as sound. Damage to the cochlea causes hearing losses that are termed sensorineural. Cochlear hearing losses result from the widest variety of causes and can occur at any age.

Objectives

1. You should know and understand the terms in the matching exercise.
2. You should be able to fill in the outline, selecting items from the list provided.
3. You should be able to label the different parts of the inner ear as shown in Figures 8A-1 and 8A-2.
4. You should be able to answer the multiple-choice questions and understand the anatomy and physiology of the inner ear as well as the causes of disorders that produce sensorineural hearing loss in the inner ear.
5. You should be able to complete the crossword puzzle.

Matching

Match the term from the column on the right with its definition.

Definition

1. ___ The efferent portion of a neuron

2. ___ A procedure designed to monitor spontaneous or induced nystagmus

3. ___ Fluid contained in the vestibular and cochlear portions of the bony labyrinth that surrounds the membranous labyrinth

4. ___ The central portion of a nerve cell

5. ___ A vascular strip along the outer wall of the scala media that supplies oxygen to the cochlea

6. ___ The cavity of the inner ear that contains the organs of equilibrium

7. ___ Nerves that carry impulses from the periphery to the brain

8. ___ Three loops within the vestibule that monitor angular acceleration

9. ___ The smaller of two sacs in the vestibule that is responsible for sensing linear acceleration

10. ___ The cochlear duct containing the organ of Corti

11. ___ The widened ends of the semicircular canals that contain the cristae

12. ___ Oscillatory movement of the eyes

13. ___ Fluid contained in the membranous labyrinth

14. ___ The membrane separating the scala media from the scala tympani and supporting the organ of Corti

15. ___ The interconnecting canals in the temporal bone that contain perilymph in which is found the membranous labyrinth

16. ___ The branching portion of a neuron that carries impulses to the cell body

Term

a. Afferent
b. Ampulla
c. Axon
d. Basilar membrane
e. Cell body
f. Cochlea
g. Dendrite
h. Efferent
i. Electronystagmography
j. Endolymph
k. Helicotrema
l. Labyrinth
m. Neuron
n. Nystagmus
o. Perilymph
p. Reissner's membrane
q. Saccule
r. Scala media
s. Scala tympani
t. Scala vestibuli
u. Semicircular canals
v. Stria vascularis
w. Tectorial membrane
x. Utricle
y. Vertigo
z. Vestibule

17. ___ The duct in the inner ear above the scala media that contains perilymph

18. ___ The larger of two sacs in the vestibule that is responsible for sensing linear acceleration

19. ___ Nerves that carry impulses from the brain to the periphery

20. ___ The sensation of true turning or spinning

21. ___ The membrane separating the scala vestibuli from the scala media

22. ___ The membrane in the scala media above the organ of Corti into which the tips of the hair cells are embedded

23. ___ The duct below the scala media that is filled with perilymph

24. ___ An opening at the apical end of the cochlea connecting the scala vestibuli with the scala tympani

25. ___ A cell specialized for conveying nerve impulses

26. ___ A cavity in the temporal bone containing the end organ of hearing

Outline

The Inner Ear

Anatomy of the Cochlea

1. _____

2. _____

3. _____

4. _____

5. _____

6. _____

7. _____

8. _____

9. _____

10. _____

11. _____

12. _____

13. _____

14. _____

Anatomy of the Vestibule

15. _____

16. _____

17. _____

18. _____

19. _____

20. _____

Disorders

21. _____

22. _____

23. _____

24. _____

Select From

A. Ampulla
B. Anoxia
C. Basilar membrane
D. Cortilymph
E. Crista
F. Drug-induced
G. Ductus reuniens
H. Hair cells
I. Helicotrema
J. Labyrinth
K. Macula
L. Méniére disease
M. Noise-induced
N. Organ of Corti
O. Otosclerosis
P. Prenatal viral infections
Q. Presbycusis
R. Postnatal viral infections
S. Reissner's membrane
T. Saccule
U. Scala media
V. Scala tympani
W. Scala vestibuli
X. Semicircular canals
Y. Skull fracture
Z. Spiral ligament
AA. Stria vascularis
AB. Tectorial membrane
AC. Utricle

25. _____

26. _____

27. _____

28. _____

29. _____

Activities

Label the parts of the labyrinth and cross section of the cochlea in the figures that follow. Select the names from the lists provided.

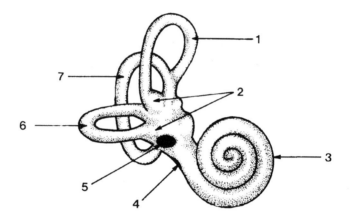

FIGURE 8A-1.   The labyrinth.

Label	*Term*
1. _____	**A.** Ampullae
2. _____	**B.** Cochlea
3. _____	**C.** Horizontal (lateral) semicircular canal
4. _____	**D.** Inferior (posterior) semicircular canal
5. _____	**E.** Oval window
6. _____	**F.** Round window
7. _____	**G.** Superior (anterior) semicircular canal

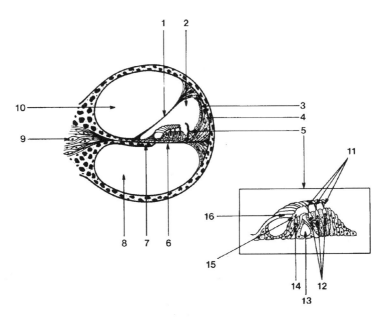

FIGURE 8A-2. **Cross section of cochlea.**

Label		*Term*
1. _____		**A.** Basilar membrane
2. _____		**B.** Inner hair cell cilia
3. _____		**C.** Inner hair cells
4. _____		**D.** Organ of Corti
5. _____		**E.** Outer hair cell cilia
6. _____		**F.** Outer hair cells
7. _____		**G.** Reissner's membrane
8. _____		**H.** Scala media (endolymph)
9. _____		**I.** Scala tympani (perilymph)
10. _____		**J.** Scala vestibuli (perilymph)
11. _____		**K.** Spiral ganglion
12. _____		**L.** Spiral lamina
13. _____		**M.** Spiral ligament
14. _____		**N.** Stria vascularis
15. _____		**O.** Tectorial membrane
16. _____		**P.** Tunnel of Corti

Multiple Choice

1. A device used to measure oscillatory movement of the eyes in response to caloric stimulation is called an
   a. electronystagmograph
   b. electroencephalograph
   c. electromyograph
   d. audiograph

2. The stria vascularis does not
   a. carry blood
   b. support hair cells
   c. produce a DC potential
   d. produce endolymph

3. The type of cerebral palsy most associated with sensorineural hearing loss is
   a. spasticity
   b. rigidity
   c. athetosis
   d. ataxia

4. Angular acceleration is measured in
   a. cm/sec^2
   b. cm/sec
   c. $degrees/sec$
   d. $degrees/sec^2$

5. The macula is the end organ located within the
   a. semicircular canals
   b. cochlea
   c. utricle
   d. brain

6. ____ does not make up a wall of the cochlear duct
   a. Bony shelf
   b. Tectorial membrane
   c. Basilar membrane
   d. Reissner's membrane

7. Endolymph is found in the
   a. stria vascularis
   b. scala vestibuli
   c. scala media
   d. scala tympani

8. The fluid surrounding the membranous labyrinth is called
   a. cortilymph
   b. perilymph
   c. endolymph
   d. lymph

9. The portion of the inner ear that responds to angular acceleration is called
   a. macula
   b. semicircular canals
   c. organ of Corti
   d. utricle

10. The central core around which the cochlea winds is the
    a. modiolus
    b. Reissner's membrane
    c. helicotrema
    d. basilar membrane

11. The tips of the outer hair cells are embedded in
    a. Reissner's membrane
    b. the bony shelf
    c. the tectorial membrane
    d. the basilar membrane

12. The most common postnatal cause of bilateral hearing loss from viral infection is
    a. rubeola (measles)
    b. rubella (German measles)
    c. pertussis (whooping cough)
    d. varicella (chicken pox)

13. Linear acceleration is measured in
    a. cm/sec^2
    b. cm/sec
    c. degrees/sec
    d. degrees/sec^2

14. Which of the following is not considered a perinatal cause of hearing loss?
    a. anoxia
    b. trauma
    c. rubella
    d. prolonged labor

15. Deprivation of oxygen, which may cause damage to the cochlea (and the brain), is called
    a. dysphemia
    b. dyscalculia
    c. dyslogia
    d. anoxia

16. The small opening allowing passage of perilymph from scala vestibuli to scala tympani is called
    a. modiolus
    b. stria vascularis
    c. spiral ligament
    d. helicotrema

17. The number of turns of the cochlea is
   a. 2
   b. 2 ½
   c. 3
   d. 3 ½
18. The structure just medial to the oval window is the
   a. cochlea
   b. semicircular canals
   c. vestibule
   d. helix
19. The crista is the end organ of the
   a. utricle
   b. saccule
   c. cochlea
   d. semicircular canals
20. Rapid back and forth movement of the eyes is called
   a. vertigo
   b. nystagmus
   c. dizziness
   d. near sightedness
21. The fluid contained in the membranous labyrinth is
   a. perilymph
   b. cortilymph
   c. blood
   d. endolymph
22. The end organ of hearing is the
   a. crista
   b. macula
   c. helicotrema
   d. organ of Corti
23. The portion of the inner ear responsible for linear acceleration is the
   a. semicircular canals
   b. utricle and saccule
   c. crista
   d. organ of Corti
24. During caloric testing when a normal left ear is stimulated with cold water, the eye beat is
   a. right
   b. left
   c. random
   d. unpredictable

25. Endolymph differs from perilymph because in endolymph
   a. potassium concentration is greater
   b. potassium concentration is less
   c. sodium concentration is greater
   d. resting microvoltage is less

26. Screening for hearing loss in the ultra-high-frequency range is often useful in detecting hearing loss caused by
   a. noise
   b. infection
   c. Méniére disease
   d. ototoxic drugs

27. Méniére disease is associated with
   a. bilateral hearing loss, good speech recognition
   b. unilateral hearing loss, poor speech recognition
   c. unilateral hearing loss, good speech recognition
   d. normal vestibular findings

28. Hereditary cochlear hearing loss resulting from genetic and environmental interactions is called
   a. homozygous
   b. hereditodegenerative
   c. multifactorial
   d. x-linked

29. Rh interactions put a baby at risk when
   a. mother is positive, father is positive
   b. mother is negative, father is negative
   c. mother is positive, father is negative
   d. mother is negative, father is positive

30. Presbycusis is hearing loss associated with
   a. aging
   b. noise
   c. bacterial infection
   d. viral infection

31. Sudden unilateral cochlear hearing loss may be caused by
   a. spasm of the internal auditory artery
   b. Méniére disease
   c. labyrinthitis
   d. all of the above

32. A hearing loss due to aging that is associated with loss of outer hair cells and supporting cells in the basal turn of the cochlea is called
   a. sensory presbycusis
   b. neural presbycusis
   c. strial presbycusis
   d. cochlear conductive presbycusis

33. Associated with cochlear hearing loss is
  a. loudness decruitment
  b. negative SISI scores
  c. loudness recruitment
  d. rapid tone decay
34. The ABR latency-intensity function for wave V expected in cochlear hearing losses is
  a. increased, primarily at high intensities
  b. increased, primarily at low intensities
  c. decreased, primarily at high intensities
  d. decreased, primarily at low intensities

Crossword

Across

2. The membrane that supports the organ of Corti

3. The branching portion of a neuron that carries impulses to the cell body

9. An opening at the apex of the cochlea that connects scala vestibuli with scala tympani

12. That part of a nerve cell that carries impulses away from the cell body

13. Nerves that carry impulses from the brain

15. The end organ of hearing in the cochlea

16. Fluid contained in the labyrinth that is high in sodium and low in potassium

17. A widened area in the semicircular canal that contains the crista

18. The membrane that separates scala vestibuli from scala media

Down

1. The organ in the vestibule responsible for horizontal linear acceleration

4. The membrane above the organ of Corti in which the tips of the outer hair cells are embedded

5. A cell designed to conduct nerve impulses

6. The interconnecting canals of the inner ear

7. The cavity of the inner ear that contains the organs of hearing

8. The portion of the vestibule responsible for vertical linear acceleration

10. The test for balance disturbances (abbr.)

11. Nerves that carry impulses to the brain

13. Fluid contained in the labyrinth that is high in potassium and low in sodium

14. An oscillating movement of the eyes

Crossword

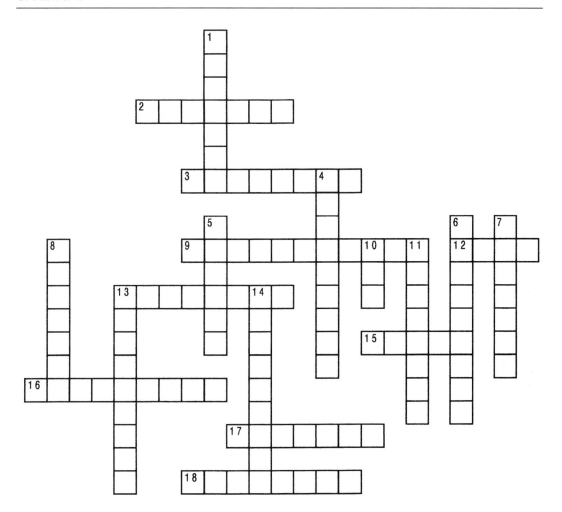

Answers—Unit A

Matching

1. c	**10.** r	**19.** h			
2. i	**11.** b	**20.** y			
3. o	**12.** n	**21.** p			
4. e	**13.** j	**22.** w			
5. v	**14.** d	**23.** s			
6. z	**15.** l	**24.** k			
7. a	**16.** a	**25.** m			
8. u	**17.** t	**26.** f			
9. q	**18.** x				

Outline

1. C	**16.** E
2. D	**17.** K
3. G	**18.** T
4. H	**19.** X
5. I	**20.** AC
6. J	**21.** B
7. N	**22.** F
8. S	**23.** L
9. U	**24.** M
10. V	**25.** O
11. W	**26.** P
12. Z	**27.** Q
13. AA	**28.** R
14. AB	**29.** Y
15. A	

Activities

Labyrinth

1. G
2. A
3. B
4. F
5. E
6. C
7. D

Cross Section of Cochlea

1. G
2. H
3. N
4. M
5. D
6. A
7. L
8. I
9. K
10. J
11. E
12. F
13. P
14. C
15. B
16. O

Multiple Choice

1. a	**14.** c	**27.** b
2. b	**15.** d	**28.** c
3. c	**16.** d	**29.** d
4. d	**17.** b	**30.** a
5. c	**18.** c	**31.** d
6. b	**19.** d	**32.** a
7. c	**20.** b	**34.** d
8. b	**21.** d	
9. b	**22.** d	
10. a	**23.** b	
11. c	**24.** a	
12. a	**25.** a	
13. a	**26.** d	

Crossword

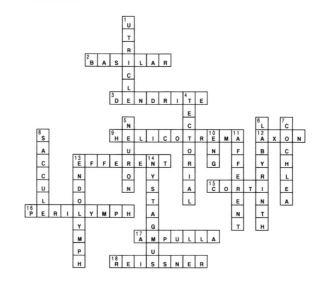

UNIT B: NOISE

Background

Some estimates show that for several years the level of noise in the environment increased by as much as a decibel a year. Since no noise in nature can threaten human hearing without being infinitely more dangerous to physical safety, it is humankind that has visited this modern epidemic upon itself. Excessive noise can interfere with communication, cause or increase hearing loss, cause nervous disorders, and it has been linked to a number of physical and psychological diseases and decreased life expectancy. Noise-induced hearing losses may be of gradual or sudden onset, the latter sometimes referred to as acoustic trauma. The audiogram typical of a noise-induced hearing loss shows the greatest deficit in the 3000- to 6000-Hz range, often showing recovery of hearing in the higher frequencies; hence, the term *acoustic trauma notch*. Those hearing losses that improve over time have been called temporary threshold shifts (TTS), and those that do not improve have been called permanent threshold shifts (PTS). The audiologist must try to discover if noise is a factor in a patient's hearing loss and then help, by counseling, to find ways of preventing progression of the loss. Many audiologists are active in the industrial, military, legal, and political arenas, where debates about noise continue to be waged.

Objectives

1. You should know and understand the terms in the matching exercise.
2. You should be able to fill in the outline, selecting items from the list provided.
3. You should know the factors in the environment that produce dangerous noise levels.
4. You should know some strategies for dealing with patients who are exposed to high noise levels, including counseling techniques and the fitting of hearing protectors.
5. You should be able to answer the multiple-choice questions on the subject of noise.
6. You should be able to complete the crossword puzzle.

Matching

Match the term from the column on the right with its definition

Definition

1. ___ Noise-induced hearing loss associated with sudden onset of intense noise

2. ___ A device that measures the intensity of noise over a period of time

3. ___ A federal agency designed to oversee the preservation of health and safety in the workplace

4. ___ Noise analysis with a sound-level meter that filters the sounds into narrow bands of 1 octave

5. ___ A reversible loss of hearing caused by intense noise

6. ___ Criteria for avoiding noise-induced hearing loss that include noise intensity and time of exposure

7. ___ An irreversible loss of hearing caused by intense noise

8. ___ Any unwanted signal

Term

a. Acoustic trauma
b. Damage-risk criteria
c. Noise
d. Noise dosimeter
e. Octave-band analysis
f. OSHA
g. Permanent threshold shift
h. Temporary threshold shift

Outline

Noise

Auditory Effects

1. _____

2. _____

3. _____

4. _____

5. _____

Select From

A Acoustic Trauma notch
B. Audiometric monitoring
C. EPA
D. Gunfire
E. Illness
F. Industry
G. Machinery
H. Muffs

Noise

Nonauditory Effects

6. _____

7. _____

8. _____

9. _____

Causes

10. _____

11. _____

12. _____

Measurement

13. _____

14. _____

15. _____

Damage-Risk Criteria

16. _____

17. _____

Agencies and Laws

18. _____

19. _____

20. _____

21. _____

Protection

22. _____

23. _____

Hearing Conservation

24. _____

25. _____

Select From

I. Nervous disorders
J. NIOSH
K. Noise abatement
L. Noise dosimeter
M. Noise exposure time
N. Noise intensity
O. Noise survey
P. OSHA
Q. PTS
R. Plugs
S. Property damage
T. Psychological disorders
U. Sensorineural hearing loss
V. Speech interference
W. Sound-level meter
X. TTS
Y. Walsh-Healey Act

Multiple Choice

1. The drop in high-frequency hearing sensitivity secondary to sudden noise exposure is often called
   a. anacusis
   b. Carhart notch
   c. otosclerosis
   d. acoustic trauma notch

2. An irreversible impairment of hearing secondary to intense noise exposure is called
   a. permanent threshold shift
   b. conductive hypacusis
   c. temporary threshold shift
   d. anacusis

3. Many patients with noise-induced hearing loss report tinnitus in the frequency area of
   a. 250 Hz
   b. 500 Hz
   c. 4000 Hz
   d. 10,000 Hz

4. Sounds that produce a noise-induced hearing loss may be
   a. uncomfortably loud
   b. painful
   c. not uncomfortably loud
   d. all of the above

5. When the A scale of a sound-level meter is used, there is
   a. maximum de-emphasis of the low frequencies
   b. moderate de-emphasis of the high frequencies
   c. slight de-emphasis of the high frequencies
   d. equal emphasis on all frequencies

6. Damage-risk criteria include the
   a. spectrum of the noise
   b. intensity of the noise
   c. duration of exposure
   d. all of the above

7. Maximum attenuation of noise is accomplished with
   a. acoustic earplugs in the ears
   b. fingers in the ears
   c. tragus pushed into the ear canal
   d. hands placed over the ears

8. Cases in which hearing thresholds improve after an initial impairment from excessive noise are called
   a. temporary threshold shift
   b. permanent threshold shift
   c. conductive hypacusis
   d. anacusis

9. The first federal act placing limits on noise levels allowable in workplaces doing government contract work was called
   a. ANSI
   b. ASA Act
   c. Walsh-Healey Act
   d. EPA Act
10. The filter setting used for most noise measurements on sound-level meters is the
    a. A scale
    b. B scale
    c. C scale
    d. D scale
11. Nonauditory effects of noise include
    a. property damage
    b. disease
    c. nervous conditions
    d. all of the above
12. A hunter who consistently fires a rifle from the right shoulder would be expected to have
    a. a greater loss in the right ear
    b. a greater loss in the left ear
    c. equal loss in both ears
    d. none of the above

Crossword

Across

4. Loss of hearing associated with sudden exposure to intense noise (2 words)
6. Any unwanted signal
7. Device used to measure sound intensity (abbr.)
8. The federal agency responsible for environmental concerns (abbr.)
9. The federal agency responsible for health and safety in the workplace (abbr.)

Down

1. The criteria by which time of safe exposure to noise are judged (2 words)
2. Device used to measure average noise exposure over time
3. An irreversible loss of hearing caused by noise (abbr.)
5. A noise-induced hearing loss that reverses spontaneously over time (abbr.)

Crossword

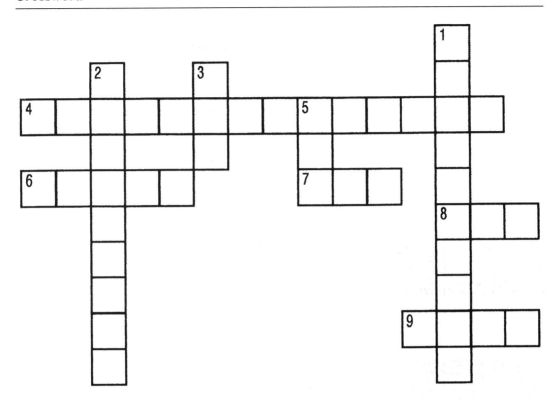

Answers—Unit B

Matching	Outline		Multiple Choice
1. a	**1.** A	**14.** O	**1.** d
2. d	**2.** Q	**15.** W	**2.** a
3. f	**3.** U	**16.** M	**3.** c
4. e	**4.** V	**17.** N	**4.** d
5. h	**5.** X	**18.** C	**4.** a
6. b	**6.** E	**19.** J	**6.** d
7. g	**7.** I	**20.** P	**7.** c
8. c	**8.** S	**21.** Y	**8.** a
	9. T	**22.** H	**9.** c
	10. D	**23.** R	**10.** a
	11. F	**24.** B	**11.** d
	12. G	**25.** K	**12.** b
	13. L		

Crossword

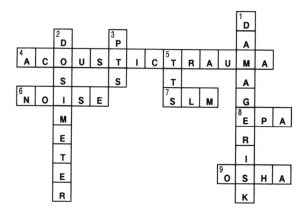

$Chapter$ 9

The Auditory Nerve and Central Auditory Pathways

Background

The nerve fibers arising from the cristae of the semicircular canals and the maculae of the utricle and saccule form the vestibular branch of the auditory (VIIIth cranial) nerve. The nerve fibers from the cochlea emerge from the modiolus to form the cochlear branch of the VIIIth nerve, which is primarily afferent (sensory) in that it carries impulses from the cochlea to the brain. It is also efferent (inhibitory), carrying impulses back to the inner ear by way of the olivocochlear bundle. The VIIIth nerve ascends to the brain stem through the internal auditory canal, from which the cochlear branch goes to a series of ipsilateral (same side of the brain) and contralateral (opposite side of the brain) waystations on its way to Heschl's gyrus in the temporal lobe. There is tonotopicity in many of these waystations.

Objectives

1. You should know and understand the terms in the matching exercise.
2. You should be able to fill in the outline, selecting items from the list provided.
3. You should be able to label the different parts of the auditory pathways in Figure 9-1.
4. You should be able to do the matching exercise.
5. You should be able to answer the multiple-choice questions and understand the anatomy of the central auditory system as well as causes of disorders that produce sensorineural hearing loss or auditory processing difficulties.
6. You should be able to complete the crossword puzzle.

Matching

Match the term from the column on the right with its definition.

Definition

1. ___ The base of the brain where it connects to the spinal cord

2. ___ The gray matter on the surface of the brain

3. ___ That part of the central auditory pathway found in the midbrain

4. ___ The area of the brain stem that provides facilitation and inhibition of afferent stimuli

5. ___ The VIIIth cranial nerve

6. ___ The area of the pons that connects the ventral cochlear nucleus with the lateral lemniscus on the other side of the brain

7. ___ The bridge connecting the two hemispheres the brain at its base

8. ___ Anatomical arrangement according to the best frequency of stimulation

9. ___ The area of the brain receiving fibers from the ipsilateral cochlea by way of the VIIIth cranial nerve

10. ___ Part of the auditory pathway receiving fibers from the cochlear nucleus

11. ___ The theory that nerve units fire their entire electrical charge when their threshold of stimulation is reached

12. ___ The superior temporal gyrus of the brain

13. ___ Fibers in the temporal cortex received from the medial geniculate body

14. ___ The addition of energy to stimulate a nerve unit

15. ___ The part of the brain above the pons and medulla that is responsible for equilibrium

16. ___ The crossing over of nerve fibers from one side of the brain to the other

Term

a. All-or-none theory
b. Auditory nerve
c. Auditory radiations
d. Brain stem
e. Central nervous system
f. Cerebellopontine angle
g. Cerebellum
h. Cerebral cortex
i. Cochlear nucleus
j. Commissure
k. Decussation
l. Excitation
m. Extra-axial
n. Glia
o. Heschl's gyrus
p. Inferior colliculus
q. Inhibition
r. Integration
s. Internal auditory canal
t. Intra-axial
u. Lateral lemniscus
v. Medial geniculate body
w. Olivocochlear bundle
x. Pons
y. Reticular formation
z. Superior olivary complex
aa. Thalamus
ab. Tonotopicity
ac. Trapezoid body

17. ___ The passage from the inner ear to the brain stem containing the two branches of the VIIIth nerve, facial nerve, and internal auditory artery

18. ___ Arresting or restraining a neural impulse

19. ___ The portion of the auditory pathway running from the cochlear nucleus to the inferior colliculus and medial geniculate body

20. ___ A group of fibers in the brain stem that provides inhibition to the cochlear nucleus and cochlea

21. ___ The brain and spinal cord

22. ___ Connective tissue in the brain

23. ___ Within the brain stem

24. ___ The combining of different neural functions to facilitate a process

25. ___ The area in the brain base that communicates with the cortex

26. ___ The last subcortical relay station, found in the thalamus

27. ___ The junction at the base of the brain where the cerebellum, medulla, and pons communicate

28. ___ Outside of the brain stem

29. ___ Specialized nerve fibers that connect the hemispheres of the brain

Outline

The Auditory Nerve and Central Pathways

Anatomy of the Vlllth Nerve

1. _____

2. _____

3. _____

4. _____

Waystations in the Brain Stem

5. _____

6. _____

7. _____

8. _____

9. _____

First-Order Neurons

10. _____

Second-Order Neurons

11. _____

Waystations in the Midbrain

12. _____

13. _____

Fibers in the Cortex

14. _____

15. _____

Disorders

16. _____

17. _____

18. _____

19. _____

20. _____

21. _____

Select From

A. Aging
B. Auditory radiations
C. Cochlea to cochlear nucleus
D. Cochlear branch
E. Course from the cochlear nucleus
F. Dorsal cochlear nucleus
G. Heschl's gyrus
H. Inferior colliculus
I. Internal auditory canal
J. Lateral lemniscus
K. Medial geniculate body
L. Multiple sclerosis
M. Myelin sheath
N. Neuritis
O. Superior olivary complex
P. Trapezoid body
Q. Trauma
R. Tumors
S. Ventral cochlear nucleus
T. Vestibular branch
U. Viral infections

Activity

Label the parts of the ascending auditory pathways in Figure 9-1, selecting the terms from the list provided. Compare your labels with those at the end of this unit.

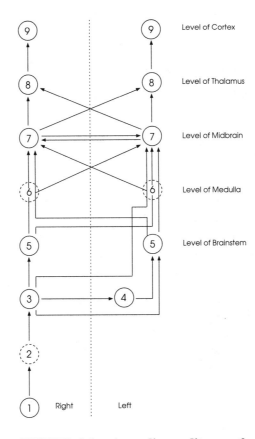

FIGURE 9-1. Ascending auditory pathways.

Label	*Term*
1. _____	**A.** Auditory cortex
2. _____	**B.** Auditory nerve (cochlear branch)
3. _____	**C.** Cochlea
4. _____	**D.** Cochlear nucleus (dorsal and ventral)
5. _____	**E.** Inferior colliculus
6. _____	**F.** Lateral lemniscus
7. _____	**G.** Medial geniculate body
8. _____	**H.** Superior olivary complex
9. _____	**I.** Trapezoid body

Multiple Choice

1. To test for central auditory disorders in a patient with normal hearing sensitivity, the audiologist will
    a. increase the extrinsic redundancy
    b. decrease the extrinsic redundancy
    c. increase the intrinsic redundancy
    d. decrease the intrinsic redundancy
2. The last subcortical relay station for auditory impulses is the
    a. inferior colliculus
    b. lateral lemniscus
    c. cochlear nucleus
    d. medial geniculate body
3. The auditory nerve is number
    a. V
    b. VI
    c. VII
    d. VIII
4. The efferent auditory system is designed for
    a. control of muscular activity
    b. feedback to lower auditory centers
    c. feed through to higher auditory centers
    d. work only at high intensities
5. The reticular formation is thought to aid in
    a. facilitation
    b. inhibition
    c. both of the above
    d. neither a nor b
6. The eyeblink is mediated through
    a. superior olivary complex
    b. inferior colliculus
    c. lateral lemniscus
    d. cochlear nucleus
7. Lesions of the central auditory nervous system include
    a. tumors
    b. degenerative diseases
    c. trauma
    d. all of the above
8. Acoustic neuromas usually form
    a. on the facial nerve
    b. on the cochlear branch of the auditory nerve
    c. on the vestibular branch of the auditory nerve
    d. in the superior olivary complex

9. Crossover points uniting symmetrical portions of the two halves of the brain are called
   a. tonotopic
   b. decussations
   c. neurons
   d. none of the above

10. Fibers cross from the left cochlear nucleus to the right cochlear nucleus via the
    a. trapezoid body
    b. superior olivary complex
    c. lateral lemniscus
    d. inferior colliculus

11. The cochlear nucleus is divided into
    a. superior and inferior portions
    b. left and right portions
    c. dorsal and ventral portions
    d. none of the above

12. Impulses are transmitted from the lower brain stem to the inferior colliculus by way of the
    a. lateral lemniscus
    b. medial geniculate body
    c. thalamus
    d. auditory radiations

13. Heschl's gyrus is located in the
    a. brain stem
    b. midbrain
    c. thalamus
    d. cortex

14. Given a patient with a lesion of the left auditory nerve, a rollover on a PI/PB function would be expected in
    a. the right ear
    b. the left ear
    c. both ears
    d. neither ear

15. Given a patient with a lesion of the left temporal lobe, a rollover on a PI/PB function would be expected in
    a. the right ear
    b. the left ear
    c. both ears
    d. neither ear

16. On auditory brain-stem response (ABR) testing a patient with a tumor of the left auditory nerve would be expected to show
    a. longer latency to wave V in the right ear than in the left ear
    b. longer latency to wave V in the left ear than in the right ear
    c. the same latency for both ears
    d. none of the above

17. Otoacoustic emissions in cases of acoustic neuroma are expected to be
    a. absent in the impaired ear, present in the normal ear
    b. present in the impaired ear, absent in the normal ear
    c. absent in the impaired ear, absent in the normal ear
    d. present in the impaired ear, present in the normal ear

Crossword

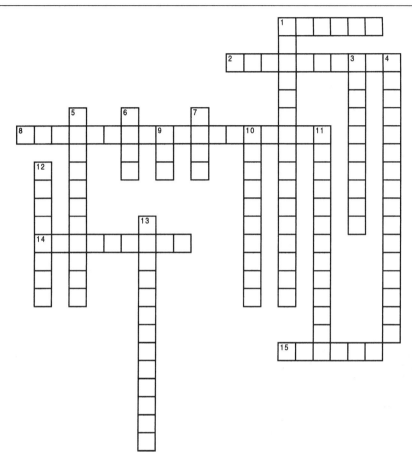

Across

1. The thin layer of gray matter on the top of the brain
2. Outside the brain stem (2 words)
8. A part of the auditory pathway found in the midbrain (2 words)
14. The formation in the brain stem designed for facilitation and inhibition of stimuli
15. The fatty sheath found on some nerve fibers

Down

1. The angle at the base of the brain where the cerebellum, medulla, and pons meet
3. Within the brain stem (2 words)
4. The auditory pathway that runs from the cochlear nucleus to the inferior colliculus (2 words)
5. The crossover of fibers from one side of the brain to the other
6. The bridge connecting the two cerebral hemispheres
7. Supporting cells of the nervous system
9. The brain and spinal cord (abbr.)
10. Special nerve fibers connecting the two hemispheres of the brain
11. Part of the auditory pathway central to the cochlear nucleus (2 words)
12. The area between the frontmost and back-most parts of the developing brain
13. A bundle of nerve units in the brain stem that sends inhibitory messages (2 words)

Answers to Chapter 9

Matching

1. d	**11.** a	**21.** e
2. h	**12.** o	**22.** n
3. p	**13.** c	**23.** t
4. y	**14.** l	**24.** r
5. b	**15.** g	**25.** aa
6. ac	**16.** k	**26.** v
7. x	**17.** s	**27.** f
8. ab	**18.** q	**28.** m
9. i	**19.** u	**29.** j
10. c	**20.** w	

Outline

1. D	**12.** H
2. I	**13.** K
3. M	**14.** B
4. T	**15.** G
5. F	**16.** A
6. J	**17.** L
7. O	**18.** M
8. P	**19.** Q
9. S	**20.** R
10. C	**21.** U
11. E	

Activity

1. C
2. B
3. D
4. I
5. H
6. F
7. E
8. G
9. A

Multiple Choice

1. b	**10.** a
2. d	**11.** c
3. d	**12.** a
4. b	**13.** d
5. c	**14.** b
6. a	**15.** a
7. d	**16.** b
8. c	**17.** a
9. b	

Crossword

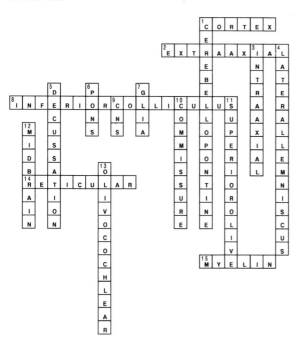

C h a p t e r ***10***

Pseudohypacusis

Background

Some patients seen for hearing evaluations may feign or exaggerate a hearing loss. Terms that describe this behavior, which may be on a conscious or unconscious level, include pseudohypacusis, nonorganic hearing loss, malingering, psychogenic hearing loss, functional hearing loss, conversion deafness, and a host of others. It is the responsibility of the audiologist to recognize pseudohypacusis and to determine the patient's true hearing status, albeit without the patient's cooperation. Some tests are quantitative; that is, they provide fairly precise information about a patient's true organic thresholds; other tests are merely qualitative and provide evidence of pseudohypacusis. After diagnosis comes the sometimes more formidable task of patient management and, when indicated, appropriate referral.

Objectives

1. You should know and understand the terms in the matching exercise.
2. You should be able to fill in the outline, selecting items from the list provided.
3. You should know which tests are appropriate for different kinds and degrees of pseudohypacusis.
4. You should know the equipment that is required for different tests for pseudohypacusis.
5. You should be able to answer the multiple-choice questions on pseudohypacusis.
6. You should be able to complete the crossword puzzle.

Matching

Match the term from the column on the right with its definition.

Definition

1. ___ A test for pseudohypacusis utilizing spondees and sawtooth noise

2. ___ The willful act of feigning a hearing loss or other disorder

3. ___ Early auditory evoked potentials

4. ___ A test for nonorganicity using Békésy audiometry with a long interval between pulsing tones

5. ___ Pseudohypacusis presumably at the unconscious level

6. ___ A test based on the fact that people speak more loudly when they hear a loud noise

7. ___ The modern term for claimed hearing loss that is not explainable in terms of organic pathology

8. ___ A test using automatic audiometry involving pulsed and continuous tones that increase and decrease in intensity

9. ___ A synonym for pseudohypacusis

10. ___ A test for pseudohypacusis involving a delay between the time a patient taps a finger or utters a word and the time the sound is heard

Term

a. Auditory brain-stem response

b. BADGE test

c. Delayed auditory feedback

d. Doerfler-Stewart test

e. Lengthened off-time test

f. Lombard test

g Malingering

h Nonorganic hearing loss

i Pseudohypacusis

j Psychogenic hearing loss

Outline

Pseudohypacusis

Terminology

1. _____

2. _____

3. _____

4. _____

5. _____

6. _____

Tests for Unilateral Pseudohypacusis

7. _____

8. _____

Tests for Bilateral Pseudohypacusis

9. _____

10. _____

General Tests for Pseudohypacusis

11. _____

12. _____

Select From

A. Auditory brain-stem response
B. Conversion deafness
C. Delayed auditory feedback
D. Doerfler-Stewart test
E. Functional hearing loss
F. Lombard test
G. Malingering
H. Nonorganic hearing loss
I. Pseudohypacusis
J. Psychogenic hearing loss
K. Stenger test
L. Swinging Story Test

Multiple Choice

1. When a nonorganic hearing loss is suspected, the audiologist may best increase cooperation by
   a. confronting the patient
   b. counseling the patient about his or her ethical responsibilities
   c. shifting the blame to the examiner
   d. insisting on greater attention to the tests
2. A nonorganic hearing loss of an unconscious nature is called
   a. sinistrosis
   b. psychogenesis
   c. pseudohypacusis
   d. malingering

3. The following is *not* an alerting sign for pseudohypacusis
    a. source of referral
    b. behavior during the interview/case history
    c. elevated acoustic reflexes
    d. performance on routine tests
4. The problem with most tests for pseudohypacusis is that they are
    a. nonqualitative
    b. nonquantitative
    c. too qualitative
    d. easy to beat
5. The following test for pseudohypacusis is limited to unilateral losses
    a. pure-tone delayed auditory feedback
    b. Stenger test
    c. Doerfler-Stewart test
    d. Lombard test
6. The following is a common type of finding with pseudohypacusis
    a. SRT worse than PTA
    b. sensorineural loss with absent acoustic reflexes
    c. conductive loss with absent acoustic reflexes
    d. lack of cross-hearing in unilateral loss
7. The Lombard test can be done as part of
    a. delayed-speech feedback
    b. Doerfler-Stewart test
    c. Swinging Story Test
    d. Stenger test
8. In pseudohypacusis the general finding is
    a. SRT = PTA
    b. SRT lower (better) than PTA
    c. SRT higher (poorer) than PTA
    d. SRT = SDT
9. The following test gives the best estimate of threshold
    a. pure-tone DAF
    b. Stenger test
    c. Doerfler-Stewart test
    d. Lombard test
10. Elevation of vocal output in the presence of noise is called the
    a. Lombard voice reflex
    b. paracusis willisi
    c. Doerfler-Stewart effect
    d. Stenger effect
11. Malingering can be proven only if
    a. the patient admits it
    b. ABR reveals normal hearing
    c. the Stenger is positive
    d. otoacoustic emissions are present

12. Pseudohypacusis involving a deliberate act is called
    a. hysterical deafness
    b. psychogenic hearing loss
    c. nonorganic hearing loss
    d. malingering
13. Threshold can probably best be determined on a pseudohypacusis patient showing bilateral hearing loss with the
    a. Swinging Story Test
    b. ABR
    c. Doerfler-Stewart test
    d. Stenger test
14. The probability of a Type V Békésy pattern is increased in patients with pseudohypacusis when
    a. duty cycle is changed to 50 percent
    b. on-time is lengthened
    c. off-time is lengthened
    d. pulsed tones are tested before continuous tones
15. Pseudohypacusis is suspected from Békésy audiometry when
    a. pulsed tones show higher (poorer) thresholds than continuous tones
    b. pulsed tones show lower (better) thresholds than continuous tones
    c. pulsed tones show the same thresholds as continuous tones
    d. none of the above
16. The minimum contralateral interference level is designed to
    a. screen for nonorganicity on the Stenger
    b. indicate precise threshold on the Stenger
    c. modify the Stenger
    d. approximate threshold on the Stenger
17. Key tapping is used with
    a. pure-tone DAF
    b. speech DAF
    c. LOCK test
    d. Békésy audiometry
18. The latest addition to the battery of tests for pseudohypacusis is
    a. otoacoustic emissions
    b. ABR
    c. Stenger test
    d. Lombard test

Crossword

Across

5. The modern term for nonorganic hearing loss

6. The lapse in time between a subject's generation of a sound and when it is heard (abbr.)

7. Auditory evoked potentials shown within the first 10 msec of stimulus presentation (abbr.)

8. A test for malingering using tones that are automatically made louder and softer (acronym)

Down

1. Nonorganic hearing loss that is not willfully produced

2. A test for malingering based on the fact that people speak more loudly in the presence of noise

3. The willful act of pretending of have a disorder (such as a hearing loss)

4. Békésy audiometry carried out with increased off-time and normal on-time (acronym)

Crossword

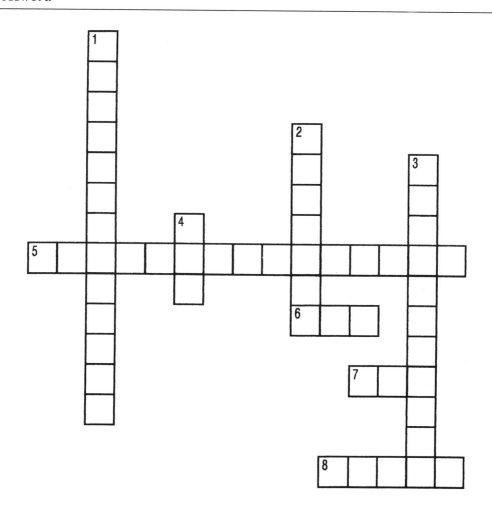

Answers to Chapter 10

Matching		*Outline*		*Multiple Choice*	
1. d	**6.** f	**1.** B	**7.** K	**1.** c	**10.** a
2. g	**7.** i	**2.** E	**8.** L	**2.** b	**11.** a
3. a	**8.** b	**3.** G	**9.** D	**3.** c	**12.** d
4. e	**9.** h	**4.** H	**10.** F	**4.** b	**13.** b
5. j	**10.** c	**5.** I	**11.** A	**5.** b	**14.** c
		6. J	**12.** C	**6.** d	**15.** a
				7. a	**16.** d
				8. b	**17.** a
				9. a	**18.** a

Crossword

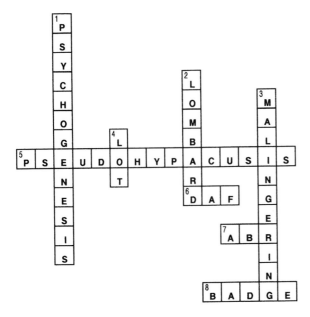

Chapter 11

The Pediatric Patient

UNIT A: PEDIATRIC DIAGNOSIS

Background

Although many young children can take adult hearing tests that have been only slightly modified, others require special procedures and special equipment. There is no argument about whether hearing loss in children should be detected as early and accurately as possible. What is in debate are the means, methods, accuracy, and cost-effectiveness of different approaches. No hearing test on a noncooperative child is foolproof, so a battery of procedures is best advised when diagnosis is critical.

Objectives

1. You should know and understand the terms in the matching exercise.
2. You should be able to fill in the outline, selecting items from the list provided.
3. You should know which hearing tests to use with children of different ages or different levels of function.
4. You should know what special equipment is necessary for specific tests.
5. You should be able to answer the multiple-choice questions on pediatric diagnosis.
6. You should be able to complete the crossword puzzle.

Matching

Match the term from the column on the right with its definition.

Definition

1. ___ A set of criteria designed to help identify infants and young children at risk for hearing loss

2. ___ A system for checking the reliability of group screening tests

3. ___ Observation of changes in the behavior of small children in response to sound

4. ___ An automated device for determining pure-tone thresholds in children

5. ___ The use of tangible reinforcement to condition young children to take a hearing test

6. ___ Use of a light or picture to reinforce a child's response to sound

7. ___ The use of games or other play techniques in teaching children to respond during hearing tests

8. ___ A sound-field hearing test for children involving localization of the sound with visual reinforcement for head turning

9. ___ Reinforcement of a child's response to a sound by illumination of a picture

10. ___ A startle response to sound in the form of an embracing movement

11. ___ Contraction of the muscles around the eyes in response to a loud sound

12. ___ A motion-sensing device that indicates when an infant has responded to a sound while lying in a crib

Term

a. Auropalpebral reflex

b. Behavioral observation audiometry

c. Conditioned orientation reflex

d. Crib-o-gram

e. High-risk register

f. Moro reflex

g. Operant conditioning audiometry

h. Pediacoumeter

i. Peep show

j. Play audiometry

k. Tetrachoric table

l. Visual reinforcement audiometry

Outline

Pediatric Diagnosis

Testing Infants

1. _____

2. _____

3. _____

4. _____

Testing Infants and Small Children

5. _____

6. _____

7. _____

Testing Small Children

8. _____

9. _____

10. _____

11. _____

Testing Older Children

12. _____

13. _____

14. _____

15. _____

16. _____

17. _____

Electrophysiological Tests

18. _____

19. _____

20. _____

Select From

A. Auditory brain-stem response
B. Auropalpebral reflex
C. Acoustic reflex threshold
D. Behavioral observation audiometry
E. Conditioned orientation response
F. Crib-o-gram
G. High-risk register
H. Moro reflex
I. Noisemakers
J. Operant conditioning audiometry
K. Pediacoumeter
L. Peep show
M. Play audiometry
N. Sound instrument test
O. Sound toy test
P. Speech-discrimination tests
Q. Speech-recognition threshold
R. Tympanometry
S. Visual response audiometry
T. Warblet

Multiple Choice

1. A motion-sensing device used in neonatal hearing testing is called
   a. crib-o-gram
   b. ABR
   c. EDR
   d. SPAR
2. Probably the easiest nonlanguage child to misdiagnose is the one with a hearing loss in
   a. the low frequencies
   b. the high frequencies
   c. the speech frequencies
   d. all frequencies
3. Difficulties encountered when using noisemakers to test neonates is control
   a. distance
   b. intensity
   c. frequency
   d. all of the above
4. The "eye blink response" from infants to loud sounds is called
   a. ABR
   b. COR
   c. Moro's
   d. APR
5. Minimum sensory deprivation syndrome may be suspected of children with
   a. repeated otitis media
   b. Rh incompatibility
   c. family history of hearing loss
   d. prematurity
6. Present thinking on neonatal screening is that it should be performed
   a. on all neonates
   b. on neonates failing one part of the high-risk register
   c. on neonates who seem not to hear
   d. on no neonates
7. Electrodermal audiometry has been largely abandoned as a test for small children because
   a. the stimuli are too noxious for most children
   b. results were often unreliable
   c. further habilitation efforts are often affected adversely because of the child's fears
   d. all of the above
8. COR utilizes
   a. one loudspeaker and one lighted doll
   b. one loudspeaker and two lighted dolls
   c. two loudspeakers and one lighted doll
   d. two loudspeakers and two lighted dolls

9. ABR has some limits in pediatric diagnosis because
   a. it does not provide information about hearing in the low frequencies
   b. it does not provide information about hearing in the high frequencies
   c. it provides information only about the speech frequencies
   d. none of the above
10. Normal speech-detection thresholds in children do not necessarily mean normal hearing because
    a. hearing may be normal only in the low- or high-frequency range
    b. they may not be able to discriminate what they hear
    c. the SRT may be lower than the SDT
    d. none of the above
11. An infant's startle response to a loud sound may mean
    a. normal hearing in both ears
    b. normal hearing in one ear
    c. a moderate hearing loss with recruitment
    d. all of the above
12. Ideally, public school hearing screening programs would include
    a. pure-tone screening
    b. pure-tone screening and tympanometry
    c. pure-tone screening, tympanometry, and acoustic reflexes
    d. pure-tone screening, tympanometry, acoustic reflexes, and SRTs
13. In operant conditioning the reinforcer should
    a. immediately follow the response
    b. be tangible
    c. be positive
    d. all of the above
14. Otoacoustic emissions have an advantage in neonatal hearing testing in that they
    a. are stable and reliable
    b. can be measured when the child is asleep or awake
    c. are unaffected by medications use to put a child to sleep
    d. all the above

Crossword

Across

3. A device using puppets as reinforcers to children's responses to tones

6. The use of a light or similar stimulus to serve as a reinforcer for a child's response (abbr.)

7. Using tangible reinforcement to encourage children's responses to sound (abbr.)

9. Criteria determined as a register to predict possible hearing loss in neonates (2 words)

Down

1. Noting activity change as an indication of a child's response to sound (abbr.)

2. A motion-sensing device in an infant's mattress to detect responses to sound (hyph.)

3. The use of pictures as a visual reinforcer to a child's response to loud sounds (2 words)

4. An eye-blink-like response to loud sounds (abbr.)

5. An embracing reflex shown by infants as a startled reaction to sound

8. A child's hearing test using localization to a light as a response to a sound (abbr.)

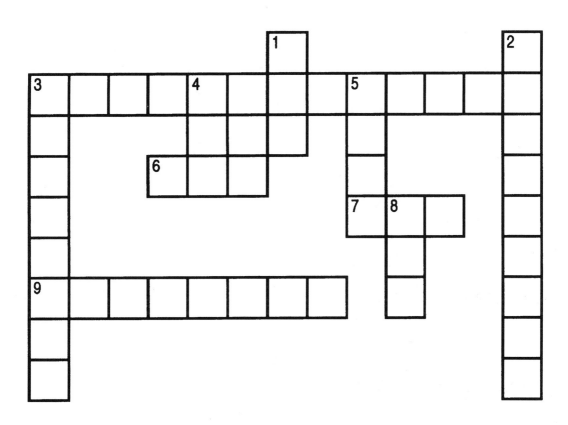

Answers—Unit A

Matching

1.	e	**7.**	j
2.	k	**8.**	c
3.	b	**9.**	i
4.	h	**10.**	f
5.	g	**11.**	a
6.	l	**12.**	d

Outline

1.	B	**11.**	S
2.	F	**12.**	J
3.	G	**13.**	K
4.	T	**14.**	L
5.	D	**15.**	M
6.	H	**16.**	P
7.	I	**17.**	Q
8.	E	**18.**	A
9.	N	**19.**	C
10.	O	**20.**	R

Multiple Choice

1.	a	**8.**	d
2.	b	**9.**	a
3.	d	**10.**	a
4.	d	**11.**	d
5.	a	**12.**	c
6.	b	**13.**	d
7.	d	**14.**	d

Crossword

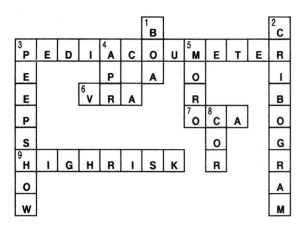

UNIT B: EDUCATION OF CHILDREN WITH HEARING IMPAIRMENTS

Background

Children who are born with or acquire a hearing loss before they develop speech and language are said to be prelinguistically hearing impaired. If their hearing loss exceeds 70 dB HL, they cannot be expected to hear more than the loudest environmental sounds and will not develop spoken language or achieve a suitable education without special training. If the loss exceeds 90 dB HL, even with amplification, the auditory channel alone will not suffice for their learning. The proper methods of educating children with a severe hearing handicap are not agreed upon, even among the most well-meaning experts. One group believes that the "deaf" should be considered as a group unto themselves with no attempt made to integrate them educationally into a hearing environment. These people are often committed to one of several forms of manual communication. The so-called "oralists" believe that children should be taught speech at all costs, taking maximum advantage of residual hearing through amplification, and should use no signs whatever. Still others believe in a combined approach of simultaneously speaking and signing. Regardless of the preferred method, there is universal agreement that the earlier the hearing loss is detected and steps taken toward educating the child, the better the prognosis for the development of language at an early age and the achievement of the highest possible educational attainment.

Objectives

1. You should know and understand the terms in the matching exercise.
2. You should be able to fill in the outline, selecting items from the list provided.
3. You should understand the methods, advantages, and disadvantages of the manual approaches to educating children with hearing impairments.
4. You should understand the methods, advantages, and disadvantages of the oral approaches to educating children with hearing impairments.
5. You should understand the methods, advantages, and disadvantages of the combined approaches to educating children with hearing impairments.
6. You should be able to answer the multiple-choice questions on pediatric management.
7. You should be able to complete the crossword puzzle.

Matching

Match the term from the column on the right with its definition.

Definition

1. ___ The use of hand signs and facial and body movements in communicating with persons with a hearing impairment

2. ___ A method of manual communication that follows English word order but is relatively uncommon

3. ___ Writing in the air with the fingers to spell out words

4. ___ Using hand signs with specific signs for articles and verbs

5. ___ A unisensory approach to teaching children with severe hearing loss that relies solely on hearing

6. ___ A less than normally rigid system of signs

7. ___ Educating individuals with hearing impairment to maximize auditory cues, often utilizing drilling exercises

8. ___ Educating children in the least restrictive environment

9. ___ A multisensory approach to teaching speech

Term

a. Acoupedic method
b. American Sign Language
c. Auditory aural
d. Auditory training
e. Finger spelling
f. Linguistics of visual English
g. Mainstreaming
h. Signing essential English
i. Signing exact English

Outline

Education of Children Who Are Hearing Impaired

Goals

1. _____

2. _____

3. _____

4. _____

5. _____

Select From

A. American Sign Language
B. Auditory global method
C. Auditory training
D. Educational achievement
E. Educational potential
F. Finger spelling
G. Integration into deaf society

Education of Children Who Are Hearing Impaired

Assessment

6. _____

7. _____

8. _____

9. _____

Communication Skills

10. _____

11. _____

12. _____

13. _____

Communication Systems

14. _____

15. _____

16. _____

17. _____

18. _____

19. _____

20. _____

21. _____

22. _____

Select From

H. Integration into hearing society
I. Intelligence
J. Language
K. Language concepts
L. Linguistics of visual English
M. Multisensory stimulation
N. Personality
O. Psychological potential
P. Seeing essential English
Q. Signing exact English
R. Social potential
S. Speech
T. Speech reading
U. Systematic sign language
V. Total communication

Multiple Choice

1. The sign system about which most information is known is
   a. ASL
   b. LOVE
   c. SEE1
   d. AMESLISH

2. All elements of English grammar may be included in
   a. LOVE
   b. SEE1
   c. finger spelling
   d. ASL

3. The least extensive sign system in terms of vocabulary is
   a. ASL
   b. LOVE
   c. SEE1
   d. SEE2

4. Signing and speaking simultaneously is called
   a. ASL
   b. total communication
   c. visual communication
   d. SEE3

5. A generic term describing hearing disability regardless of degree is
   a. hearing impaired
   b. hard of hearing
   c. deaf
   d. deafened

6. Children with hearing losses in the 70- to 90-dB HL range may be expected to
   a. have difficulty mainly with faint speech
   b. understand conversation at distances less than 5 feet
   c. understand speech only if speakers raise their voices
   d. identify loud sounds near the ear and perhaps a few vowel sounds

7. Given appropriate training and amplification, success may usually be achieved in regular schools by children with hearing losses up to
   a. 30 dB HL
   b. 50 dB HL
   c. 70 dB HL
   d. 90 dB HL

8. Early identification is most likely for a child with a hearing loss of
   a. 20 dB HL
   b. 40 dB HL
   c. 60 dB HL
   d. 80 dB HL

9. The acoupedic method of training children who have hearing impairments
   a. insists on auditory cues exclusively
   b. insists on visual cues exclusively
   c. combines visual with auditory cues
   d. none of the above
10. Public Law 94-142 mandates that
    a. all handicapped children must be educated in regular classrooms
    b. all children who have hearing impairments must be educated in regular classrooms
    c. all children must be educated in the least restrictive environment
    d. children with hearing losses greater than 90 dB HL must be educated in special classrooms
11. The Auditory Global Method states that
    a. the exclusive teaching channel should be auditory
    b. the primary teaching channel should be auditory
    c. the primary teaching channel should be visual
    d. the same teaching methods should be used all over the world
12. Many experts feel that integration of a child with hearing impairment into a regular classroom is best achieved with a teaching method involving
    a. finger spelling
    b. signing
    c. auditory-oral
    d. none of the above
13. The intelligence of young children who have severe hearing impairments is best determined by tests that
    a. rely heavily on language
    b. rely lightly on language
    c. rely heavily on performance
    d. include finger spelling for instruction
14. Assessing personality in young children who cannot hear is difficult because
    a. tests are complicated by vocabulary items
    b. personality development is related closely to language development
    c. emotional immaturity is caused by frustration in some children
    d. all of the above
15. Teaching children who cannot hear to speak involves senses that are
    a. tactile
    b. kinesthetic
    c. visual
    d. all of the above
16. Children who are prelinguistically hearing impaired are not those who
    a. lose hearing shortly after birth
    b. are born with hearing loss
    c. lose hearing before they learn language
    d. lose hearing after they learn language

17. Teaching systems for children who cannot hear that include vision, hearing, tactile, and kinesthetic senses are called
    a. unisensory
    b. acoupedic
    c. multisensory
    d. ASL
18. Auditory training may take advantage of
    a. a wearable hearing aid
    b. a magnetic loop system
    c. an FM carrier system
    d. all of the above
19. Speech-reading is usually taught to children
    a. in isolation
    b. in combination with other lessons
    c. without amplification
    d. in darkened areas to increase concentration
20. Many experts agree that children with hearing losses sufficient to require hearing aids should be fitted
    a. when the child can care for the instrument
    b. at the age when children normally begin to speak
    c. at the earliest possible time regardless of age
    d. when the child reaches school age

Crossword

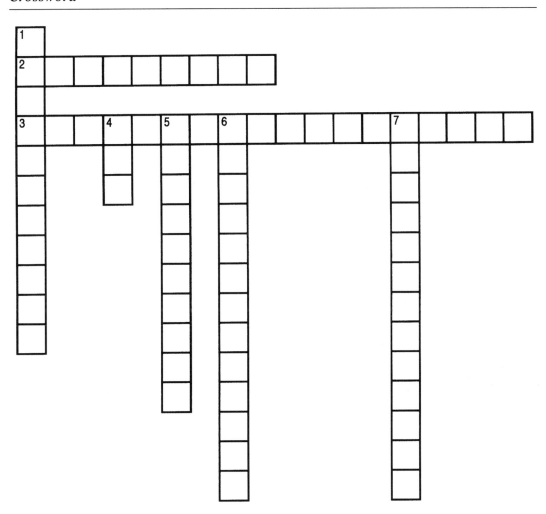

Across

2. A unisensory approach to children with hearing loss, depriving them of visual stimulation

3. Using speech and signs together to teach speech to children with hearing loss (2 words)

Down

1. Finger-spelling

4. Ameslan (abbr.)

5. The use of hand shapes near the mouth to facilitate speech reading

6. Educating children with handicaps in the least restrictive environment

7. Multisensory stimulation for teaching children with hearing loss (2 words)

Answers—Unit B

Matching

1.	b	**6.**	i
2.	f	**7.**	d
3.	e	**8.**	g
4.	h	**9.**	c

Outline

1.	E	**12.**	S
2.	G	**13.**	T
3.	H	**14.**	A
4.	O	**15.**	B
5.	R	**16.**	F
6.	D	**17.**	L
7.	I	**18.**	M
8.	K	**19.**	P
9.	N	**20.**	Q
10.	C	**21.**	U
11.	J	**22.**	V

Multiple Choice

1.	a	**11.**	b
2.	c	**12.**	c
3.	b	**13.**	c
4.	b	**14.**	d
5.	a	**15.**	d
6.	d	**16.**	d
7.	d	**17.**	c
8.	d	**18.**	d
9.	a	**19.**	b
10.	c	**20.**	c

Crossword

Chapter 12

Management of Hearing Impairment

UNIT A: APPROACHES TO REHABILITATION

Background

All the diagnostic audiological information gathered on a patient is useless unless it translates into some form of constructive action that helps the patient to communicate. Medical or surgical reversal of hearing loss is preferable, but when this is impossible or when the treatment does not result in sufficient functional hearing, steps must be taken to improve the patient's communicative abilities by utilizing residual hearing. High on the list of measures to be considered is the selection and training in the use of proper hearing aids if this is feasible. Other measures include auditory (re)training; speech reading; and, foremost, education and counseling of patients and their families regarding the implications of hearing loss. Although drill work in speech reading or discrimination of sounds is still widely practiced, it is considered by many clinicians not to be the most effectual means of audiological rehabilitation for many persons. Many clinicians today construct their therapy around hearing-handicap scales, completed by the patient, to help to judge the kinds of communicative difficulties that are experienced. Proper audiological rehabilitation is the culmination of the efforts of the clinical audiologist.

Objectives

1. You should know and understand the terms in the matching exercise.
2. You should be able to fill in the outline, selecting items from the list provided.
3. You should try to understand some of the feelings of many patients with hearing disabilities so that these may be dealt with more efficiently.

4. You should understand the basic principles of speech-reading training.
5. You should understand the basic principles of auditory training.
6. You should understand the basic principles of patient counseling.
7. You should be able to answer the multiple-choice questions.
8. You should be able to complete the crossword puzzle.

Matching

Match the term from the column on the right with its definition.

Definition

1. ___ A class of closely related speech sounds

2. ___ The production of speech as it appears on the lips

3. ___ The reeducation of individuals who have lost their hearing in listening for specific auditory cues

4. ___ The use of facial cues to determine the words of a speaker

5. ___ The recording of all background information related to a hearing loss

6. ___ A ringing or other sound heard in the ears or the head

7. ___ Any part of a word that conveys meaning

Term

a. Auditory retraining
b. History taking
c. Morpheme
d. Phoneme
e. Speech reading
f. Visime
g. Tinnitus

Outline

Aural Rehabilitation

Hearing Aids

1. _____
2. _____
3. _____
4. _____
5. _____

Select From

A. Adjustment to hearing aid
B. Analytical methods
C. Combining with residual hearing
D. Group counseling
E. Group hearing aid
F. Individual counseling

Aural Rehabilitation	***Select From***

Speech Reading

6. _____

7. _____

8. _____

9. _____

Auditory Training

10. _____

11. _____

12. _____

14. _____

Counseling

15. _____

16. _____

17. _____

G. Individual hearing aids
H. Hearing aid evaluation
I. Hearing aid orientation
J. Social strategies
K. Word recognition in noise
L. Word recognition in quiet
M. Synthetic methods
N. Tolerance for loud sounds
O. Training in noise
P. Training in quiet
Q. Visible phonemes

Multiple Choice

1. Hearing aids should be selected for patients based on
   a. the hearing loss in the better ear
   b. the hearing loss in the poorer ear
   c. the average hearing loss in both ears
   d. individual hearing needs
2. Least important in the selection of hearing aids is
   a. freedom from internal noise
   b. quality of sound
   c. shape
   d. intelligibility provided for faint words
3. Important to a course in auditory training is the teaching of
   a. discrimination among speech sounds
   b. discrimination of speech sounds from nonspeech sounds
   c. discrimination of sound from silence
   d. all of the above

4. Speech detection implies
   a. sensing whether a sound is present
   b. the nature of a particular sound
   c. discrimination among speech sounds
   d. all of the above

5. Identification of speech sounds by a patient may be indicated by
   a. repeating the sound
   b. pointing to a picture or item
   c. writing down what was heard
   d. all of the above

6. Auditory retraining is a term used to denote that
   a. the hearing loss was adventitious
   b. the hearing loss was congenital
   c. the hearing loss was inherited
   d. all of the above

7. Audiological rehabilitation is usually most difficult for a patient with a moderate hearing loss that is
   a. conductive
   b. mixed
   c. sensorineural
   d. unilateral

8. The term *habilitation* is usually used when describing work with
   a. very young children
   b. teenagers
   c. adults
   d. the elderly

9. Aural rehabilitation often involves teaching adults to
   a. utilize contextual cues in speech
   b. make reasonable guesses
   c. predict language patterns
   d. all of the above

10. The least difficult listening situation for the new hearing-aid wearer is
    a. understanding in quiet places
    b. understanding in noisy places
    c. understanding rapid speakers
    d. understanding unusual vocabulary

11. Patients wearing hearing aids can learn to improve the signal-to-noise ratio when listening in a noisy place by
    a. raising the volume of the hearing aids
    b. moving closer to the speaker
    c. asking the speaker to talk louder
    d. b and c

12. A basic assumption that may be made when hearing aids are provided to a small child is that
    a. speech will be clearer
    b. speech will be louder
    c. speech will be louder and clearer
    d. visual cues are unnecessary

13. A first step in an audiological habilitation program with a small child is sound
    a. repetition
    b. awareness
    c. discrimination
    d. production

14. Although there is some disagreement, most clinicians believe that audiological habilitation should include
    a. visual cues alone
    b. auditory cues alone
    c. visual and auditory cues combined
    d. none of the above

15. Of the more than 40 phonemes used in English discourse, approximately ____ are clearly visible
    a. 90 percent
    b. 20 percent
    c. 33 percent
    d. 5 percent

16. Most difficult to speech-read are
    a. vowels
    b. consonants
    c. words in context
    d. sentences

17. Many audiologists believe that speech-reading ability
    a. can be taught equally to all patients
    b. is a talent possessed more by some people than by others
    c. is unimportant if properly fitted hearing aids are used
    d. is easily learned

18. The ability to speech-read is affected by
    a. the available light
    b. distance from the speaker
    c. rate of the speech
    d. all of the above

19. It is important to teach visual memory when teaching speech reading because
    a. speech is usually not repeated
    b. speech is rapid
    c. speech sounds, once seen, cannot be reviewed
    d. all of the above

Crossword

Across

2. The part of a word that conveys meaning
5. Teaching listening skills to patients with acquired hearing loss
6. Ringing, roaring, or other sounds in the ears
7. Use of facial cues or lip movements in understanding a speaker

Down

1. Acquisition of relevant background information on a patient
3. A class of speech sounds
4. Speech production as it appears on the lips

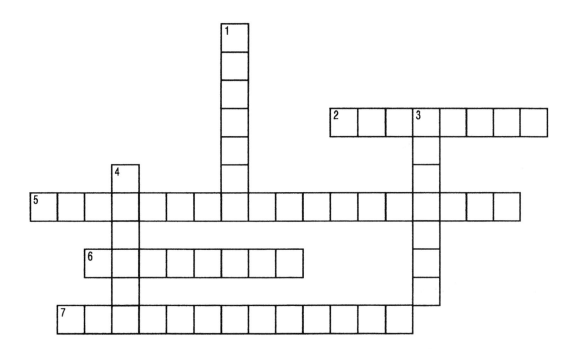

Answers—Unit A

Matching

1. d		**5.** b	
2. f		**6.** g	
3. a		**7.** c	
4. e			

Outline

1. A		**10.** K	
2. E		**11.** L	
3. G		**12.** N	
4. H		**13.** O	
5. I		**14.** P	
6. B		**15.** D	
7. C		**16.** F	
8. M		**17.** J	
9. Q			

Multiple Choice

1. d		**11.** d	
2. c		**12.** b	
3. d		**13.** b	
4. a		**14.** c	
5. d		**15.** c	
6. a		**16.** a	
7. c		**17.** b	
8. a		**18.** d	
9. d		**19.** d	
10. a			

Crossword

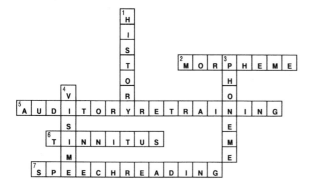

UNIT B: HEARING AIDS

Background

As the hearing aid evolved from mechanical amplifiers such as ear trumpets into the electronic era, research has focused on miniaturization, wearability, and improved sound quality. The current infusion of microprocessing techniques into the design characteristics and selection procedures for hearing aids is bringing about a new revolution in this most important aspect of auditory rehabilitation. The hearing aid is essentially a one-way transmission system containing a microphone as an input transducer, a miniature loudspeaker as an output transducer, and stages of amplification with volume control and signal shaping between these two. The system is powered by a small battery. Although there is some limited need today for bone-conduction receivers, most instruments generate air-conduction signals, which are usually delivered to the external auditory canal by a custom-made plastic ear mold. Acoustic characteristics of hearing aids are usually described in terms of their saturation sound-pressure level (SSPL) (the maximum power output that can be delivered regardless of the strength of the input signal), acoustic gain (the difference in decibels between the input and output sound-pressure levels), and the frequency response (range and output of frequencies amplified). No modern audiology clinic should be without a hearing-aid testing system that can measure the characteristics of an aid, including distortion products. Although no single procedure for evaluating and selecting the "best" hearing aids to suit an individual patient is agreed upon, the present trend is toward dispensing the selected instruments directly to the patient rather than writing a prescription for a particular make, model, and set of internal and external settings, as was popular only a short time ago. It is hoped that the days of selecting hearing aids from mail-order catalogues, or drug or department stores, are nearly over and that hearing aids can be offered to patients as part of a larger package of auditory (re)training, speech reading, hearing-aid orientation, and counseling.

Objectives

1. You should know and understand the terms in the matching exercise.
2. You should be able to fill in the outline, selecting items from the list provided.
3. You should know and be able to identify the components of a hearing aid.
4. You should understand the implications of assistive listening devices.
5. You should be able to answer the multiple-choice questions about hearing instruments.
6. You should be able to complete the crossword puzzle.

Matching

Match the term from the column on the right with its definition.

Definition

1. ___ A device surgically placed in the inner ear for persons with profound hearing loss

2. ___ The squeal that occurs when sound that is amplified and fed through the speaker of a hearing aid is picked up again by the microphone and reamplified

3. ___ The testing of several hearing instruments in the sound field to determine the most suitable one for a patient

4. ___ A device that amplifies sound and delivers it to the surface of the skin so that the different patterns of vibration can be felt

5. ___ Measurements made of sound-pressure level in the ear canal that show the performance characteristics of a hearing aid

6. ___ Signaling or alerting devices, in addition to hearing aids, that assist individuals with a hearing loss

7. ___ An electromagnetic device in a hearing aid that allows the user to bypass the microphone when talking on the telephone

8. ___ Hearing aids worn in both ears

9. ___ The highest sound pressure that can emit from a hearing aid regardless of the input intensity

10. ___ The custom-made device, usually made of plastic, that couples a hearing aid to the ear

11. ___ A system for limiting the sound intensity emitted by a hearing aid by using electronic feedback circuits

12. ___ Connection to the space between an ear mold and tympanic membrane so that a sound developed in that space can be transduced for measurement

Term

a. Acoustic feedback
b. Acoustic gain
c. Assistive listening devices
d. Automatic gain control
e. Binaural hearing aids
f. Cochlear implants
g. Compression amplification
h. Ear mold
i. Frequency response
j. Harmonic distortion
k. Hearing-aid evaluation
l. Probe tube
m. Real-ear measurements
n. Reference test gain
o. Saturation sound-pressure level
p. Telecoil
q. Vibrotactile hearing aid

13. ___ The range from the lowest to the highest frequency amplified by a hearing aid

14. ___ The increase of the intensity of a sound produced by a hearing aid as measured in a hearing-aid test box

15. ___ The difference, in decibels, between the input intensity and the output intensity of a hearing aid

16. ___ Distortion in a hearing aid produced by the generation of overtones

17. ___ Another term for automatic gain control

Outline

Hearing Aids

Types

1. _____
2. _____
3. _____
4. _____
5. _____
6. _____
7. _____
8. _____

Characteristics

9. _____
10. _____
11. _____
12. _____
13. _____
14. _____
15. _____

Select From

A. Air conduction
B. Amplifier
C. Battery
D. Behind the ear
E. Body-worn
F. Bone conduction
G. Cord
H. CROS
I. Ear mold
J. Earphone
K. Eyeglass
L. Frequency response
M. Gain
N. Harmonic distortion
O. Intermodulation distortion
P. In the canal
Q. In the ear
R. Microphone
S. Peak clipping
T. Ringing
U. SSPL
V. Telephone pickup
W. Tone control
X. Volume control

Hearing Aids

Components

16. _____

17. _____

18. _____

19. _____

20. _____

21. _____

22. _____

23. _____

24. _____

Multiple Choice

1. The maximum sound-pressure level emitted from the receiver of a hearing aid, regardless of its input level is called
   a. acoustic gain
   b. SSPL
   c. frequency response
   d. distortion
2. The difference, in decibels, between the input and the output SPL of a hearing aid is its
   a. acoustic gain
   b. SSPL
   c. frequency response
   d. distortion
3. A sweep frequency audio oscillator is used to determine a hearing aid's
   a. acoustic output
   b. SSPL
   c. frequency response
   d. distortion
4. Lack of sound coming from a hearing aid may be caused by
   a. occluded ear mold
   b. twisted tubing
   c. a broken receiver
   d. all of the above
5. Acoustic feedback will not be caused by
   a. a loosely fitting ear mold
   b. a twisted cord
   c. a loose connection between ear mold and receiver
   d. an improperly inserted ear mold

6. Weak but audible sound coming from a hearing aid will not be caused by a
   a. partially obstructed ear mold
   b. weak battery
   c. switch set to "telephone" setting
   d. partially obstructed tubing

7. The input transducer of a hearing aid is its
   a. battery
   b. microphone
   c. loudspeaker
   d. volume control

8. "Ceramic," "magnetic," "dynamic," and "electret" are different kinds of
   a. loudspeakers
   b. hearing aids
   c. microphones
   d. volume controls

9. De-emphasis of different portions of the freqaring aid may be accomplished by
   a. ear-mold modification
   b. internal tone adjustments
   c. changing receivers
   d. all of the above

10. Bone-conduction hearing aids are usually reserved for patients who have
    a. sensorineural hearing loss
    b. conductive hearing losses caused by otosclerosis
    c. conductive hearing losses with chronic ear drainage
    d. mixed hearing losses without chronic ear drainage

11. Acoustic feedback problems with hearing aids will not be lessened by
    a. cupping a hand behind the aided ear
    b. increasing the distance from microphone to receiver
    c. fabricating a tighter ear mold
    d. improving the connection between ear mold and receiver

12. The transient nature of speech can cause a hearing aid's
    a. harmonic distortion
    b. intermodulation distortion
    c. ringing
    d. acoustic feedback

13. Persons with total unilateral hearing losses are sometimes helped by a hearing aid called
    a. CROS
    b. IROS
    c. NITTS
    d. ROSS

14. A type of hearing aid that lessens the boomy sound listeners hear when they speak is
    a. ITE
    b. BTE
    c. CIC
    d. ITC

Crossword

Across

2. Comprehension amplification (abbr.)
6. The range from the lowest to the highest frequency delivered by a hearing aid (2 words)
9. Signaling or alerting devices used by patients in addition to or instead of hearing aids (abbr.)
11. The difference between the input and output levels of a hearing aid
12. Listening with both ears
13. Squeal heard from a hearing aid when the microphone is too close to the receiver
14. An electromagnetic device in a hearing aid for use with the telephone

Down

1. Device designed to amplify speech so that its vibrations can be felt on the skin
3. Device placed surgically into the inner ear to help patients with profound hearing loss (2 words)
4. Device used for real-ear measurements of a hearing aid (2 words)
5. Listening with one ear
7. Device used to couple a hearing aid to the ear
8. The highest intensity that can leave a hearing aid regardless of the input (abbr.)
10. Any unwanted sound in an amplification system

Crossword

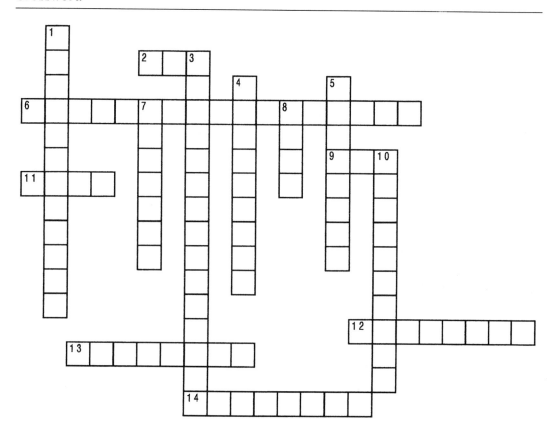

Answers—Unit B

Matching

1.	f	**10.**	h
2.	a	**11.**	d
3.	k	**12.**	l
4.	q	**13.**	i
5.	m	**14.**	n
6.	c	**15.**	b
7.	p	**16.**	j
8.	e	**17.**	g
9.	o		

Outline

1.	A	**13.**	S
2.	D	**14.**	T
3.	E	**15.**	U
4.	F	**16.**	B
5.	H	**17.**	C
6.	K	**18.**	G
7.	P	**19.**	I
8.	Q	**20.**	J
9.	L	**21.**	R
10.	M	**22.**	V
11.	N	**23.**	W
12.	O	**24.**	X

Multiple Choice

1.	b	**8.**	c
2.	a	**9.**	d
3.	c	**10.**	c
4.	d	**11.**	a
5.	b	**12.**	c
6.	c	**13.**	a
7.	b	**14.**	c

Crossword

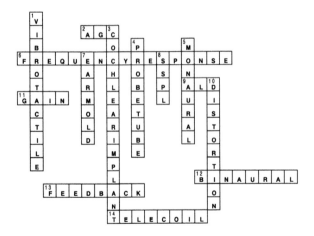

Part II

Case Studies

Case 1

History

Your patient is a 26-year-old female with a complaint of diminished hearing "for several years" that "seems to be getting worse." Her mother has told you that the patient experienced ear infections as a small child, but the patient herself has no memory of this. She has increased difficulty hearing while chewing but seems, to her surprise, to understand speech better in a noisy background than in quiet places. The patient has two older sisters with hearing losses that began in early adulthood. One wears a hearing aid successfully and the other was helped by surgery, the nature of which the patient does not know. She, along with members of her family, has a bluish cast to the whites of her eyes. Given the audiometric data on the following page and this history, make your diagnosis and substantiate it.

Diagnosis

Type of Loss   Right: _____   Left: _____

Probable Etiology

_____

Case Management

_____

_____

_____

_____

Reasons for Decision

_____

_____

_____

_____

_____

Case 1   *Audiometric Data*

Test	Right Ear	Left Ear
SRT	25 dB HL	35 dB HL
WRS	98%	100%
ARTs (ipsilateral)	Absent	Absent
ARTs (contralateral)	Absent	Absent
Static compliance	0.7 cc	0.65 cc
ABR	All waves prolonged; Interwave latencies normal; Latency-intensity function normal	All waves prolonged; Interwave latencies normal; Latency-intensity function normal
TEOAE	Absent	Absent
SISI at 4000 Hz	0%	5%
Tone decay test	0 dB of decay in 60 seconds	5 dB of decay in 60 seconds
Békésy type	I	I

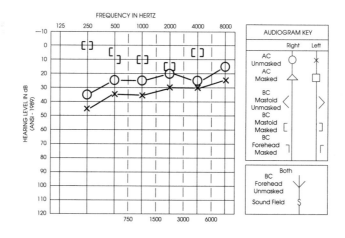

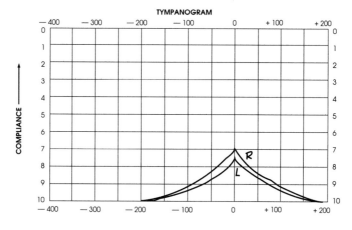

Case 1   Correct Diagnosis

Type of Loss
   Right: Conductive
   Left: Conductive

Probable Etiology
   Bilateral otosclerosis

Case Management
Refer to an otologist with a good track record doing stapedectomies. Include all audiometric data and a report stating your suspicions. Request a letter to learn the otologic diagnosis and proposed treatment.

Reasons for Decision
The normal bone conduction, air-bone gaps, and excellent word recognition scores all indicate a conductive hearing loss. The tympanograms are Type A_S in both ears, and crossed and uncrossed acoustic reflexes are absent at the limits of the equipment, suggesting middle-ear disorders. Static compliance is normal and does not assist in diagnosis. The low-frequency tilt of the audiogram suggests stiffness in the middle-ear system. The Carhart notch suggests otosclerosis, along with the family history of females with progressive hearing loss, blue sclera, paracusis willisii, and deprecusis. All special tests are consistent with a conductive hearing loss. The infections as a child have no bearing because the hearing loss had its onset years after the infections had ceased. Because one sister was helped by surgery and the other did well with hearing aids (suggesting good speech discrimination), it is likely that they too have otosclerosis.

Notes

History

Your patient is a 39-year-old male with a history of sudden hearing loss in the right ear and vertigo. Previous to an incident several months earlier, the patient had no difficulty with either hearing or balance. The course of symptoms is described as follows: The patient noted a sensation of fullness in his right ear for several days along with some slight difficulty understanding through that ear over the telephone. On the next day he noticed a humming noise in that ear followed by a loud roaring sound. He suddenly had the sensation of whirling and was unable to keep his balance; he became ill and vomited several times. He now feels that he has no hearing in his right ear although the spinning sensation has completely disappeared. Both his parents had difficulty hearing when they became much older. His greatest communication difficulty is in group situations or when people speak softly to him on his right side. Given the audiometric findings on the following page and this history, make your diagnosis and substantiate it.

Diagnosis

Type of Loss   *Right:* _____   *Left:* _____

Probable Etiology

_____

Case Management

_____

_____

_____

Reasons for Decision

_____

_____

_____

Case 2 **Audiometric Data**

Test	Right Ear	Left Ear
SRT	70 dB HL	5 dB HL
WRS	34%	100%
ARTs at 2000 Hz (ipsilateral)	85 to 95 dB HL	80 to 90 dB HL
ARTs at 4000 Hz (contralateral)	85 to 95 dB HL	80 to 90 dB HL
Static compliance	0.9 cc	0.79 cc
ABR	All waves prolonged; Interwave latencies normal; Latency-intensity function for wave V steep	All waves normal; Interwave latencies normal; Latency-intensity function for wave V normal
TEOAE	Absent	Absent
SISI at 4000 Hz (20 dB SL)	100%	0%
ABLB	Recruitment	——
Tone decay test	15 dB of decay in 60 seconds	5 dB of decay in 60 seconds
Békésy type	II	I

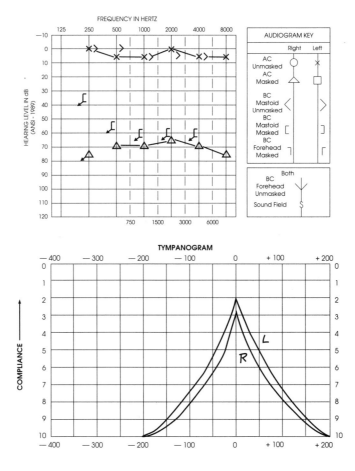

Case 2 *Correct Diagnosis*

Type of Loss
  Right: Sensorineural (Cochlear)
  Left: Normal hearing

Probable Etiology
  Unilateral Méniére disease

Case Management
Refer to an otologist with comments on your suspicions and recommend electronystagmography. If you can perform ENG in your clinic, check on its advisability before doing the test. Request a report from the physician and arrange for the patient to return for further counseling and longitudinal testing to monitor for fluctuation or progression.

Reasons for Decision
The roaring tinnitus and full aural sensations are part of the usual prodroma of Méniére disease, probably caused by increased endolymphatic pressure. All of the special tests suggest a cochlear site of lesion. The word-recognition score is extremely poor in the right ear. *All* tests in the right ear should have been performed with masking in the left ear. The presence of acoustic reflexes at normal hearing levels (low sensation levels in the right ear), along with the steep ABR latency-intensity function and absent TEOAEs suggests a cochlear disorder. The hearing losses experienced by the patient's parents do not bear on the diagnosis because they are probably caused by aging. The difficulty hearing in groups is typical of severe unilateral losses. Because hearing is normal in the left ear, the patient relies on it and is unaware of the residual hearing in the right ear.

Notes

Case 3

History

Your patient is a 34-month-old male who is brought to you by his parents. They are not certain whether a hearing loss is present, although the child says "huh" a good deal. The father believes that he "does not pay attention." The child has been "slightly behind" his two older, normal siblings (a boy and a girl) in his language development milestones. A pediatrician has treated the child with antibiotics for "ear infections" on a few occasions but more often for "tonsillitis." No marked temperature elevations were associated with these episodes, and the child is otherwise healthy. There is no family history of hearing loss, although his father has difficulty understanding speech in groups and has a constant high-pitched tinnitus since serving two years in the artillery. The child tired quickly before all the desired hearing tests could be completed, but given history and the limited audiometric data on the following page, make your diagnosis and substantiate it.

Diagnosis

Type of Loss   *Right:* _____   *Left:* _____

Probable Etiology

_____

Case Management

_____
_____
_____
_____

Reasons for Decision

_____
_____
_____
_____

Case 3   *Audiometric Data*

Test	Right Ear	Left Ear
SRT	20 dB HL	25 dB HL
WRS	?	?
Acoustic reflexes (ipsilateral)	Absent	Absent
Acoustic reflexes (contralateral)	Absent	Absent
Static compliance	0.25 cc	0.20 cc
ABR	All waves prolonged; Interwave latencies normal; Latency-intensity function normal	All waves prolonged; Interwave latencies normal; Latency-intensity function normal
TEOAE	Absent	Absent

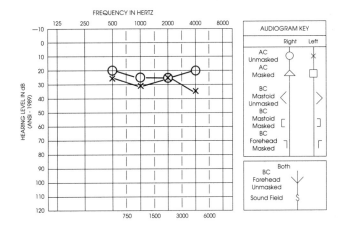

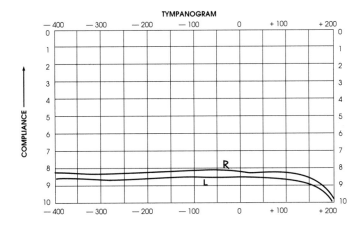

Case 1   Correct Diagnosis

Type of Loss
    Right: Conductive
    Left: Conductive

Probable Etiology
    Bilateral serous effusion

Case Management
Refer to an otologist with all your findings and suspicions. Make an appointment for further audiometric study, especially bone conduction. Request a report of the physician's findings. Stress to the parents the importance of a complete audiometric examination after all medical and/or surgical treatment has been completed. If hearing is normal upon the return visit, consider referring to a speech-language pathologist to test for language delay secondary to sensory deprivation. Suggest that the father consider a hearing evaluation for a diagnosis of his hearing problem.

Reasons for Decision
The agreement between the SRT and pure-tone average makes the diagnosis of mild hearing loss likely. The fact that the child did not take the bone-conduction test and the lack of word-recognition scores makes it impossible to state with certainty that the hearing loss is purely conductive (hence the need for further testing); however, the Type B tympanogram, the absent acoustic reflexes, low static compliance, and flat audiometric configuration all suggest fluid in the middle ear. Because there was no ear drainage, pain, or fever in the history, it is more likely that the hearing loss is due to serous effusion than to active infection. This, of course, must be determined medically. The father's hearing loss is acquired, probably because of noise, and is irrelevant to the diagnosis of the child's problem.

Notes

Case 4

History

Your patient is a 23-year-old male who was referred by his attorney for routine hearing tests because of a gradual hearing loss in his left ear associated with noise. The patient is a construction worker. There is no history of ear infections, vertigo, or tinnitus, and no reported family members with hearing loss. The patient claims that he is "totally deaf" in the left ear and requests that you write a letter to this effect "to whom it may concern." He claims that he cannot hear people speak at all when they are on his left side. Given the history and the audiometric data on the following page make your diagnosis and substantiate it.

Diagnosis

Type of Loss   *Right:* _____   *Left:* _____

Probable Etiology

_____

Case Management

_____
_____
_____
_____
_____

Reasons for Decision

_____
_____
_____
_____
_____

Case 4 *Audiometric Data*

Test	Right Ear	Left Ear
SRT	5 dB HL	NR
WRS	100%	NR
ART at 1000 Hz (ipsilateral)	95 dB HL	Absent
ART at 1000 Hz (contralateral)	85 dB HL	Absent
Static compliance	0.62 cc	0.66 cc
ABR	All waves normal; Interwave latencies normal; Latency-intensity function normal	All waves normal; Interwave latencies normal; Latency-intensity function normal
TEOAE	Present	Present

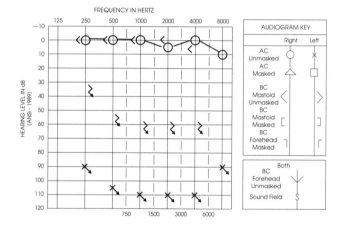

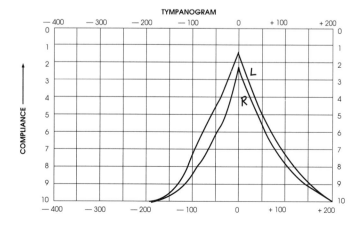

Case 4   *Correct Diagnosis*

Type of Loss
    Right: Normal hearing
    Left: Normal hearing

Probable Etiology
    Pseudohypacusis (probably malingering)

Case Management
Prepare a report in detail outlining your reasons for suspecting pseudohypacusis and the tests that support diagnosis. Retain and carefully file all test forms or paper readouts for easy retrieval. Explain to the patient that his test results are inconsistent but that you believe the hearing in his left ear to be normal or near normal. Write a letter to his attorney stating the same thing. Do not use the word "malingering." Suggest re-evaluation.

Reasons for Decision
The first tip-off to nonorganicity was the obvious lack of a shadow curve on the audiogram. If the left ear truly had a total loss, the air-conduction and speech recognition thresholds would have been about 50~0 dB (average interaural attenuation) and the bone-conduction thresholds no worse than about 15 dB. Word recognition scores obtained at high levels in the "deaf" ear should approach 100 percent as the opposite (normal) ear should respond. The normal levels at which acoustic reflexes were elicited with stimulation to the left ear prove that a total hearing loss is impossible. The Stenger test's minimum contralateral interference level of 35 dB in the left ear shows that the tone was heard loud enough at that level to make a tone in the right ear at 10 dB inaudible. Further special tests should have been performed as time allowed. High on the list of desirable tests would be the Stenger, using spondaic words and several different frequencies; the pure-tone DAF; and the SPAR test. Existing evidence for nonorganic hearing loss is clear, and malingering is likely because of the involvement of an attorney and potential lawsuit, but psychogenesis cannot be ruled out with certainty. If the hearing loss was truly caused by noise, it would have been less severe and bilateral in nature. Remember that you cannot legally release your findings or impressions to another party without express written permission by the patient.

Notes

Case 5

History

Your patient is a 42-year-old right-handed male who complains of a high-pitched ringing in his ears, which is louder and more prolonged after noise exposure than had formerly been the case. He is fond of deer and duck hunting and enjoys listening to rock music under earphones. His two sisters have progressive hearing losses that began in their 20s and seemed to get worse during pregnancy. The patient is uncertain whether he has a hearing loss per se but notices that speech often sounds muffled, and he has difficulty hearing in groups or in background noise. He has never had ear infections. Given the history and the audiometric data on the following page make your diagnosis and substantiate it.

Diagnosis

Type of Loss   *Right:* _____   *Left:* _____

Probable Etiology

_____

Case Management

_____

_____

_____

_____

_____

Reasons for Decision

_____

_____

_____

_____

_____

Case 5   *Audiometric Data*

Test	Right Ear	Left Ear
SRT	15 dB HL	25 dB HL
WRS	100%	100%
ART at 1000 Hz (ipsilateral)	85 dB HL	90 dB HL
ART at 4000 Hz (contralateral)	95 dB HL	90 dB HL
Static compliance	0.52 cc	0.65 cc
ABR	All waves prolonged; Interwave latencies normal; Latency-intensity function steep	All waves prolonged; Interwave latencies normal; Latency-intensity function steep
TEOAE	Absent	Absent
SISI at 4000 Hz	100%	100%
Tone decay test at 4000 Hz	5 dB of decay in 60 seconds	5 dB of decay in 60 seconds
Békésy type	II	I

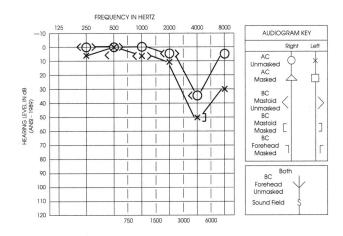

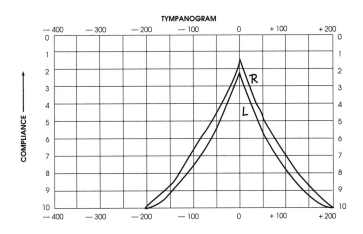

Case 5   *Correct Diagnosis*

Type of Loss
   Right: Sensorineural (cochlear)
   Left: Sensorineural (cochlear)

Probable Etiology
   Exposure to high noise levels

Case Management
Explain to the patient the nature of the loss and why the cause is probably noise. Encourage abstention from or minimizing exposure to noise. Suggest the use of hearing protectors either in the form of plugs or muffs. If possible fit the plugs yourself and/or provide the patient with precise information on where foam plugs can be obtained and their approximate cost. Encourage lower levels when listening to music and the use of loudspeakers rather than earphones. Arrange for reevaluation of hearing in six months and stress the importance of checking for progression of the loss.

Reasons for Decision
The audiogram shows the typical acoustic trauma notch; note that the loss at 4000 Hz is greater in the left ear, which is typical of persons firing a rifle from the right shoulder. The family history sounds like otosclerosis although you cannot be certain of that, and is unrelated to the patient's problem. It is likely that the patient experiences some increased loss of hearing and tinnitus immediately after noise exposure, both of which had been recovering to a greater extent in the past until the threshold shifts became more permanent. It is also likely that the patient himself realizes that noise is a probable cause of his difficulty, based on his own subjective impressions and his history.

Notes

Case 6

History

Your patient is a 16-year-old female with a lifelong history of ear infections. She reports having had mastoidectomies on both sides. A strong pungent odor is noticeable near her ears. There is no family history of hearing loss. She claims that her hearing fluctuates, at times appearing to be near normal and at other times creating severe problems in communication. She has tried a hearing aid in her right ear but constant drainage made its use impossible. She has since lost the aid. Her family doctor has told her that nothing can be done to improve her hearing and has her on a renewable prescription for ear drops. Given the case history and the audiometric data on the following page, make your diagnosis and substantiate it.

Diagnosis

Type of Loss   Right: _____   Left: _____

Probable Etiology

_____

Case Management

_____

_____

_____

_____

_____

Reasons for Decision

_____

_____

_____

_____

_____

Case 6   *Audiometric Data*

Test	Right Ear	Left Ear
SRT	45 dB HL	40 dB HL
WRS	92%	94%
Acoustic reflexes (ipsilateral)	Absent	Absent
Acoustic reflexes (contralateral)	Absent	Absent
Static compliance	NO SEAL	NO SEAL
ABR	All waves prolonged; Interwave latencies normal; Latency-intensity function normal	All waves prolonged; Interwave latencies normal; Latency-intensity function normal
TEOAE	Absent	Absent
SISI at 4000 Hz	90%	90%
Tone decay test	0 dB of decay in 60 seconds	5 dB of decay in 60 seconds
Békésy type	I	I

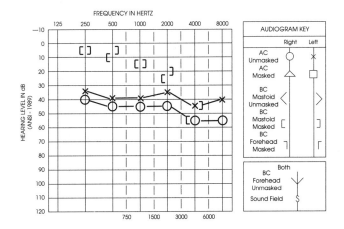

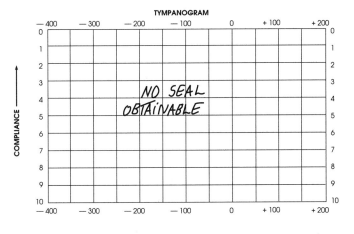

Case 6   Correct Diagnosis

Type of Loss
     Right: Mixed
     Left: Mixed

Probable Etiology
     Chronic otitis media

Case Management
Discuss with the patient her type of hearing loss she has and its relationship to her history of infections, and suggest that she consider a second opinion by an otologist. If she agrees to this referral, provide a detailed report to the otologist and request a letter with his or her diagnosis and plan for therapy. Discuss the possibility of a hearing aid in the event that the patient decides not to pursue medical treatment or if there is no evidence that treatment will result in short-term improvement in hearing. Obtain written medical clearance before proceeding with a hearing-aid evaluation and, if the ear drainage is a persistent problem, consider a bone-conduction aid. Arrange for periodic monitoring of the hearing loss and keep the patient informed of her progress. See that the patient understands the implications of the sensorineural portion of her hearing loss and recognizes that, although her hearing may be improved considerably, it cannot be made completely normal.

Reasons for Decision
The air-bone gap, high word-recognition scores, and drop in bone-conduction sensitivity in the high frequencies all indicate a mixed loss that is predominantly conductive. The cochlear reserve may actually be better than the bone-conduction thresholds indicate because of alterations in the inertial mode of bone conduction caused by the middle-ear disorder, although the high SISI scores at 4000 Hz indicate sensorineural involvement. Auditory evoked potentials and otoacoustic emissions are consistent with the cochlear portion of the hearing loss. The inability to obtain a seal upon immittance testing and the large c_1 values suggest tympanic membrane perforations, which should have been visible upon otoscopic examination prior to testing. The strong odor at the ears suggests the possibility of cholesteatomas. Diplomacy is necessary in making the new referral so that your comments will not be construed as critical of the family doctor, although surely this consultation may be necessary.

Notes

History

Your patient is a 51-year-old male who complains of vague difficulty in understanding speech, especially in noisy or otherwise untoward listening circumstances. He has no history of ear disease, skull trauma, balance difficulties, or noise exposure. Sometimes he feels that his understanding is improved if he pays very close attention. He has been seen for medical examination and no explanation for his difficulty was offered, although you are not certain of the extent of this examination. Given the history and the audiometric data on the following page, make your diagnosis and substantiate it.

Diagnosis

Type of Loss   *Right:* _____   *Left:* _____

Probable Etiology

_____

Case Management

_____

_____

_____

_____

_____

Reasons for Decision

_____

_____

_____

_____

_____

Case 7   *Audiometric Data*

Test	Right Ear	Left Ear
SRT	0 dB HL	5 dB HL
WRS	98%	100%
ART at 4000 Hz (ipsilateral)	85 dB HL	90 dB HL
ART at 4000 Hz (contralateral)	Absent	Absent
Static compliance	0.72 cc	0.80 cc
ABR	All waves normal; Interwave latencies normal; Latency-intensity function normal	All waves normal; Interwave latencies normal; Latency-intensity function normal
TEOAE	Present	Present
SISI at 4000 Hz	0%	5%
Tone decay test	0 dB of decay in 60 seconds	5 dB of decay in 60 seconds
Békésy type	I	I

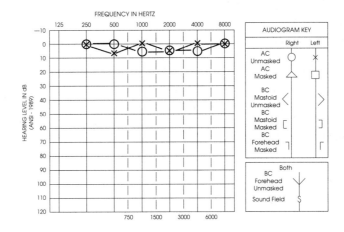

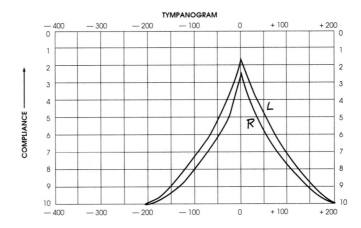

Case 7   Correct Diagnosis

Type of Loss
    Right: Normal sensitivity
    Left: Normal sensitivity

Probable Etiology
    Unknown; possible brain-stem lesion

Case Management
Reschedule the patient for a complete battery of special tests for central auditory disorders to include PI-PB functions, SSI-ICM, SSI-CCM, staggered spondaic words, and others available. Tell the patient that his difficulty is not in sounds being loud enough because the audiogram indicates normal hearing for pure tones. Explain that additional stress will have to be placed on his word recognition ability to determine the extent of his difficulty beyond what can be derived from testing with PB word lists. Discuss referral to a neurologist, which would best be done after more complete audiometric studies have been completed.

Reasons for Decision
The normal hearing sensitivity, with the kinds of complaints the patient makes, alerts you to a possible central disorder. Present ipsilateral acoustic reflexes at normal levels indicate normal middle ears and acoustic pathways, including VIIth nerve integrity, short of the crossover pathways in the brain stem. Absent contralateral acoustic reflexes suggest that the crossover pathways are involved. Low scores on the modified SISI also suggest a central lesion. More definitive testing should help in the diagnosis, but a neurological referral is imperative in any case.

Notes

Case 8

History

Your patient is a 19-year-old female college student. Her main complaint is a hearing loss that presents more difficulty in hearing and understanding speech than in hearing environmental sounds. She has had this difficulty as long as she can remember and does not believe it is getting worse. There are no known family members with a hearing loss, and she has never had any ear infections, nor has she worn hearing aids. The patient's speech is quite intelligible but there is some distortion in the production of her sibilant sounds, and her vocal tone is rather monotonous. She managed to get good grades in high school, but now that she is in college she finds school much more difficult and believes it is because of her hearing problem. You notice that she speaks rather loudly. Given the history and the audiometric data on the following page make your diagnosis and substantiate it.

Diagnosis

Type of Loss   Right: _____   Left: _____

Probable Etiology

_____

Case Management

_____
_____
_____
_____

Reasons for Decision

_____
_____
_____
_____

Case 8   *Audiometric Data*

Test	Right Ear	Left Ear
SRT	45 dB HL	40 dB HL
WRS	86%	82%
ART at 1000 Hz (ipsilateral)	90 dB HL	95 dB HL
ART at 4000 Hz (contralateral)	90 dB HL	90 dB HL
Static compliance	0.80 cc	0.78 cc
ABR	All waves prolonged; Interwave latencies normal; Latency-intensity function steep	All waves prolonged; Interwave latencies normal; Latency-intensity function steep
TEOAE	Absent	Absent
SISI at 4000 Hz	100%	100%
Tone decay test	10 dB of decay in 60 seconds	15 dB of decay in 60 seconds
Békésy type	II	II

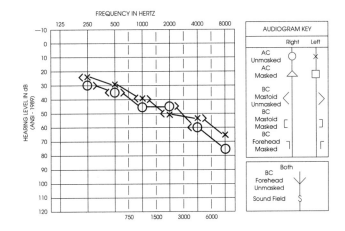

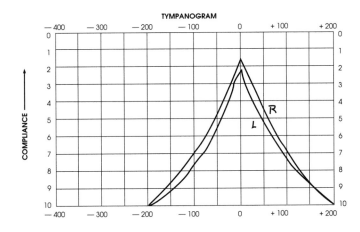

Case 8   *Correct Diagnosis*

Type of Loss
  Right: Sensorineural (probably cochlear)
  Left: Sensorineural (probably cochlear)

Probable Etiology
  Unknown; possibly congenital

Case Management
Discuss with the patient the possibility of a hearing-aid evaluation, trial period with hearing aids, and a period of auditory rehabilitation and hearing-aid orientation. Ascertain that the patient understands the nature of her hearing loss. Try to make an appointment for earmold fitting and hearing-aid tests before the patient loses interest. Arrange for medical consultation prior to making earmolds if this is required in your state. Try to make a positive yet realistic appraisal of the patient's potential for hearing-aid use. If she wishes medical consultation on the irreversibility of her hearing loss, offer to provide your findings to the physician of her choice. Check with the physician on possible blood studies and inquire about her interest in genetic counseling. If she is not interested in audiological rehabilitation at this time, suggest that she have annual reevaluations of her hearing.

Reasons for Decision
The absent air-bone gaps and diminished word-recognition scores, along with the normal tympanograms, indicate sensorineural hearing loss. The low sensation level acoustic reflexes and high SISI scores suggest a cochlear site of lesion. There is simply not enough information in the history to hazard more than a guess about the cause of the loss. The fact that the patient does not know of family members with hereditary hearing loss does not mean that there have been none. The loss may also have been acquired at an early age, caused by some disease.

Notes

$$C \ a \ s \ e \quad 9$$

History

Your patient is a 58-year-old female with a complaint of hearing loss in her right ear. The difficulty was first noticed about five years earlier and has been gradually progressive to the point where she relies for communication entirely on her left ear. She does not experience true vertigo, but frequently she has attacks of unsteadiness and occasional headaches. She also complains of a constant noise in her right ear, which she describes as "bacon frying." Her family physician has told her that the hearing loss is related to several episodes of middle-ear infection that she had as a child. Her main communication problem is in groups or noisy backgrounds, which she attempts to avoid. Given this history and the audiometric data on the following page, make your diagnosis and substantiate it.

Diagnosis

Type of Loss   *Right:* _____   *Left:* _____

Probable Etiology

_____

Case Management

_____
_____
_____
_____
_____

Reasons for Decision

_____
_____
_____
_____
_____

Case 9   *Audiometric Data*

Test	Right Ear	Left Ear
SRT	50 dB HL	5 dB HL
WRS	6%	100%
ART at 500 Hz (ipsilateral)	Absent	85 dB HL
ART at 500 Hz (contralateral)	Absent	80 dB HL
Reflex decay to half amplitude at 500 Hz	3 seconds	10+ seconds
Static compliance	0.80 cc	0.83 cc
ABR	All waves prolonged after; Wave I; Wave I to III latency increased; Latency-intensity function shallow	All waves normal; Interwave latencies increased; Latency-intensity function normal
TEOAE	Present	Present
ABLB	Decruitment	—
Modified SISI at 4000 Hz	0%	100%
Tone decay test	30 + dB of decay in 60 seconds	5 dB of decay in 60 seconds
Békésy type	III	I

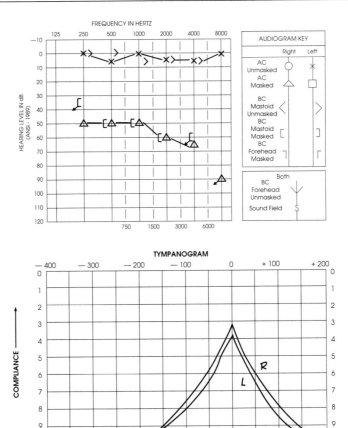

Case 9   *Correct Diagnosis*

Type of Loss
> *Right*: Sensorineural (probably neural)
> *Left*: Normal

Probable Etiology
> Acoustic neuroma

Case Management
Make a prompt referral, if possible, to a neuro-otologist or to an otologist with experience in dealing with neural lesions in the auditory tract. Detail all your findings and advise him or her that the history and auditory findings are consistent with a possible retrocochlear lesion. You may discuss your feelings about a possible lesion of the VIIIth nerve but should hesitate to put it into a report that is leaving your clinic. Short of frightening the patient, do all you can to see that the referral is followed through. Request that the physician send you results of ENG and radiologic studies, along with the diagnosis and proposed treatment.

Reasons for Decision
The left ear is completely normal on all tests and the right ear shows a moderate loss by both air and bone conduction. SRTs agree nicely with the pure-tone averages, but the word-recognition scores are extremely poor in the right ear for a moderate loss, and first raise suspicions of a retrocochlear lesion. The tinnitus is also not of the usual variety described by patients with cochlear pathology. Abnormal ABRs, present TEOAEs, loudness decruitment, marked tone decay, negative SISI scores, and Type III Békésy tracings all fit with a neural lesion in the right ear. The gradual progressive nature of the loss, the type of dizziness, and the headaches all call for an immediate referral to confirm or deny the presence of a space-occupying lesion. The history of ear infections is unrelated to the present hearing loss.

Notes

History

Your patient is an 82-year-old man with a history of gradually progressive hearing loss in both ears over the past fifteen years. He is brought, reluctantly, to the clinic by his daughter-in-law, who complains privately that "he does not pay attention." He claims that sometimes he hears better than at other times and compliments you on the fact that you are easier to understand than most people. He has tried several hearing aids, which were useless to him; he has no desire to purchase any more hearing aids. Because he finds listening in groups difficult, he has ceased attending church, parties, and the theater. He claims that people do not speak clearly and that he understands better when they speak more slowly. Given the history and the audiometric data on the following page, make your diagnosis and substantiate it.

Diagnosis

Type of Loss   Right: _____   Left: _____

Probable Etiology

Case Management

Reasons for Decision

Case 10 *Audiometric Data*

Test	Right Ear	Left Ear
SRT	50 dB HL	45 dB HL
WRS	62%	58%
ART at 1000 Hz (ipsilateral)	95 dB HL	95 dB HL
ART at 2000 Hz (contralateral)	90 dB HL	Absent
Static compliance	0.92 cc	0.65 cc
ABR	All waves normal at high SLs; Interwave latencies normal; Latency-intensity function steep	All waves normal at high SLs; Interwave latencies normal; Latency-intensity function steep
TEOAE	Absent	Absent
SISI at 4000 Hz	90%	85%
Tone decay test	10 dB of decay in 60 seconds	15 dB of decay in 60 seconds
Békésy type	II	II

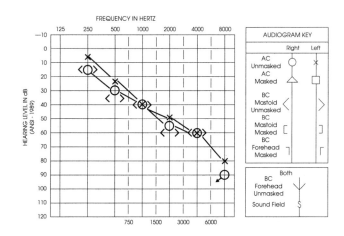

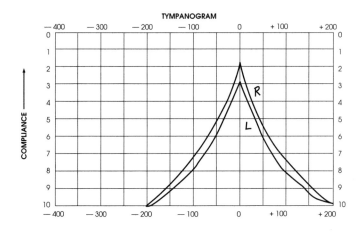

Case 10   *Correct Diagnosis*

Type of Loss
   Right: Sensorineural
   Left: Sensorineural

Probable Etiology
   Presbycusis

Case Management
Discuss the possibility of amplification for a trial period. In counseling the family, make sure that you speak directly to the patient, although the daughter-in-law should be present. Listen carefully to his complaints and do not provide more information on the nature of the hearing loss than the patient seems to desire. Advise the family that hearing aids should not be purchased until it has been demonstrated that they are of value, and that this cannot really be achieved unless the patient enrolls for a period of auditory rehabilitation that emphasizes coping strategies. Suggest the possibility of assistive listening devices, such as a personal FM system, TV hookup, and telephone amplifier. Be as reassuring as possible, short of making an unethical guarantee that the hearing loss will not progress significantly. Arrange for periodic reevaluations and, if the patient agrees, for ear-mold fabrication. If state law requires medical concurrence before proceeding, explain this to the family and assist in the arrangements.

Reasons for Decision
All immittance and audiometric results rule out any conductive hearing loss. The lack of an air-bone gap and the relatively poor word recognition all fit with a diagnosis of sensorineural hearing loss. Note that the SRT is slightly poorer than the pure-tone average; this is observed in many elderly patients. Since there is nothing specific in the history to suggest a cause for the hearing loss, it is likely that the patient's advanced age is the etiologic factor. Improved understanding of slower speech, sometimes called "phonemic regression," is sometimes seen in presbycusic patients. Convincing the patient to give hearing aids one more try will not be easy and should not be approached strenuously. This may come about if the patient feels a sense of confidence in you as an audiologist.

Notes

History

Your patient is a 39-year-old female who complains of a sudden hearing loss following an automobile accident in which her car was struck from the rear. She also claims dizziness, severe bitemporal headaches, nausea, and "blackout spells." She did not mention tinnitus until asked about it during the history taking. There is no reported family history of hearing loss, ear infections, or other symptoms that the patient now claims to experience. She requests that a written report of your findings be sent to her for her "records."

Diagnosis

Type of Loss   *Right:* _____   *Left:* _____

Probable Etiology

_____

Case Management

_____

_____

_____

_____

_____

Reasons for Decision

_____

_____

_____

_____

_____

Case 11 Audiometric Data

Test	Right Ear	Left Ear
SRT	30 dB HL	35 dB HL
WRS	86%	80%
ART at 1000 Hz (ipsilateral)	85 dB HL	85 dB HL
ART at 2000 Hz (contralateral)	80 dB HL	85 dB HL
Static compliance	0.70 cc	0.73 cc
ABR	All waves normal; Interwave latencies normal; Latency-intensity function normal	All waves normal; Interwave latencies normal; Latency-intensity function normal
ABR Wave V Threshold	15 dB HL	20 dB HL
TEOAE	Present	Present
Békésy type	V	V

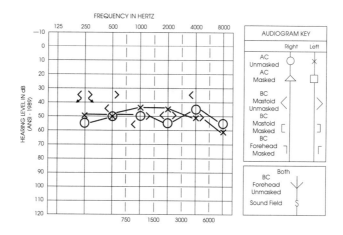

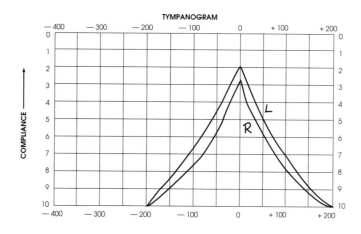

Case 1   ***Correct Diagnosis***

Type of Loss
> *Right*: Pseudohypacusis
> *Left*: Pseudohypacusis

Probable Etiology
> Possible malingering

Case Management
Complete as many tests for pseudohypacusis as time allows. Counsel the patient regarding her inconsistencies and accept the responsibility yourself for not having properly instructed her in taking the tests. Readminister the audiogram and SRT tests if time permits and arrange for rescheduling. Carefully record all your findings in a report and file carefully. Do not confront the patient or act accusatory in any way. State in a separate report to her that inconsistencies preclude diagnosis and do not mention special tests for pseudohypacusis.

Reasons for Decision
The main indicator of nonorganicity in this case is the obvious discrepancy between the SRT and the pure-tone average for each ear (the former obtained at considerably lower hearing levels) and the normal acoustic reflexes. Normal ABR results and present TEOAEs suggest normal hearing in both ears. The history itself should have alerted you to possible nonorganicity since the patient may wish to bring suit for damages against the owner of the car that struck hers, but this is not evidence in itself. The primary behavioral tests for you to perform are pure-tone delayed auditory feedback, and ascending-descending threshold exploration.

Notes

Case 12

History

Your patient is a seven-year-old female who failed the public school hearing screenings on two occasions. The child's parents have had her examined by an otologist, who could find no explanation for the apparent high-frequency hearing loss and has referred her to you for further study. The child denies any difficulty in hearing.

Diagnosis

Type of Loss   Right: _____   Left: _____

Probable Etiology

_____

Case Management

_____

_____

_____

_____

_____

Reasons for Decision

_____

_____

_____

_____

_____

Case 12 *Audiometric Data*

Test	Right Ear	Left Ear
SRT	15 dB HL	20 dB HL
WRS	100%	100%
ART at 1000 Hz (ipsilateral)	90 dB HL	90 dB HL
ART at 4000 Hz (contralateral)	85 dB HL	95 dB HL
Static compliance	0.62 cc	0.59 cc
ABR	All waves normal; Interwave latencies normal; Latency-intensity function normal	All waves normal; Interwave latencies normal; Latency-intensity function normal
TEOAE	Present	Present

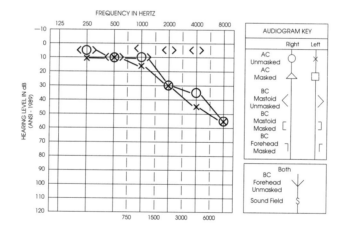

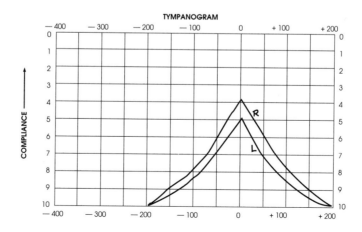

Case 12   *Correct Diagnosis*

Type of Loss
   Right: Normal hearing
   Left: Normal hearing

Probable Etiology
   Collapsing ear canals

Case Management
Retest the child with an insert receiver, a stock ear mold or plastic tubing in the ear canal to keep the canal open. If normal hearing is demonstrated, explain to the parents what has occurred and that failing the hearing test was no fault of the child. You may demonstrate to the parents how the canal collapses by placing an empty earphone cushion over the ear and allowing them to see the effect of ear canal closure through the opening. Send a letter to the referring physician with the correct audiogram and explanation of your findings.

Reasons for Decision
The high-frequency conductive hearing loss first seen in the absence of positive otological findings and the presence of normal tympanograms and acoustic reflexes are the main indications of collapsing ear canals. It is fairly easy to guess what happened in this case, but the same phenomenon can occur in the presence of a hearing loss, making diagnosis quite obscure. Careful examination at the time of otoscopy, preceding immittance measures, should alert you to possible collapsing canals. ABR and TEOAE results using insert earphones assist in the diagnosis of normal hearing.

Notes